Gender and Genetics

Prenatal screening for genetic disorders is becoming an increasingly widespread phenomenon across the globe. While studies have highlighted the importance of women's experiences of such screening, little is known about men's roles and direct involvement in this process. With a focus on the experiences of both women and men, this text offers an innovative and passionate account of the gendered nature of prenatal screening.

Drawing on interview data with pregnant women and their male partners in a UK city, Reed provides a compelling analysis of maternal and paternal roles in prenatal screening. Through this analysis, the book raises important issues around genetics, gender and screening practice. With a focus on the gendered production of 'good' and 'bad' genes, the book explores differences between visual technologies and blood screening. It also explores the gendered nature of genetic responsibility and the impact this has on parenting roles.

Extending its arguments into other key debates in prenatal genetics – including a focus on the impact of screening on other types of stratification, including ethnicity and class – Reed provides an original and comprehensive analysis of some of the most pressing concerns in the field to date. This book will be of interest to students and scholars of the sociology of health and illness, science and technology studies, gender studies, feminist bioethics and medical anthropology, as well as professionals in the fields of midwifery and genetic counselling.

Kate Reed is a senior lecturer in Medical Sociology at the University of Sheffield. She has published broadly across the areas of ethnicity, gender, social theory and the sociology of health and illness. She is the author of *Worlds of Health* (Praeger 2003) and *New Directions in Social Theory: Race, Gender and the Canon* (Sage 2006).

Genetics and society

Series Editors: Ruth Chadwick, *Director of Cesagen, Cardiff University*, John Dupré, *Director of Egenis, Exeter University*, David Wield, *Director of Innogen, Edinburgh University*, and Steve Yearley, *Director of the Genomics Forum, Edinburgh University.*

The books in this series, all based on original research, explore the social, economic and ethical consequences of the new genetic sciences. The series is based in the Cesagen, one of the centres forming the ESRC's Genomics Network (EGN), the largest UK investment in social-science research on the implications of these innovations. With a mix of research monographs, edited collections, textbooks and a major new handbook, the series is a valuable contribution to the social analysis of developing and emergent bio-technologies.

Series titles include:

New Genetics, New Social Formations
Peter Glasner, Paul Atkinson and Helen Greenslade

New Genetics, New Identities
Paul Atkinson, Peter Glasner and Helen Greenslade

The GM Debate
Risk, politics and public engagement
Tom Horlick-Jones, John Walls, Gene Rowe, Nick Pidgeon, Wouter Poortinga, Graham Murdock and Tim O'Riordan

Growth Cultures
Life sciences and economic development
Philip Cooke

Human Cloning in the Media
Joan Haran, Jenny Kitzinger, Maureen McNeil and Kate O'Riordan

Local Cells, Global Science
Embryonic stem cell research in India
Aditya Bharadwaj and Peter Glasner

Handbook of Genetics and Society
Paul Atkinson, Peter Glasner and Margaret Lock

The Human Genome
Chamundeeswari Kuppuswamy

Community Genetics and Genetic Alliances
Eugenics, carrier testing and networks of risk
Aviad E. Raz

Neurogenetic Diagnoses. The Power of Hope and the Limits of Today's Medicine
Carole Browner and H. Mabel Preloran

Debating Human Genetics
Contemporary issues in public policy and ethics
Alexandra Plows

Genetically Modified Crops on Trial
Opening up alternative futures of Euro-agriculture
Les Levidow

Creating Conditions
The making and remaking of a syndrome
Katie Featherstone and Paul Atkinson

Genetic Testing
Accounts of autonomy, responsibility and blame
Michael Arribas-Allyon, Srikant Sarangi and Angus Clarke

Regulating Next Generation Agri-Food Bio-Technologies
Lessons from European, North American and Asian experiences
Edited by Michael Howlett and David Laycock

Regenerating Bodies
Tissue and cell therapy in the twenty-first century
Julie Kent

Gender and Genetics
Sociology of the prenatal
Kate Reed

Forthcoming titles include:

Scientific, Clinical and Commercial Development of the Stem Cell
From radiobiology to regenerative medicine
Alison Kraft

Barcoding Nature
Claire Waterton, Rebecca Ellis and Brian Wynne

Negotiating Bioethics
The Governance of UNESCO's Bioethics Programme
Adèle Langlois

Gender and Genetics

Sociology of the prenatal

Kate Reed

Routledge
Taylor & Francis Group
LONDON AND NEW YORK

First published 2012
by Routledge
2 Park Square, Milton Park, Abingdon, Oxon, OX14 4RN

Simultaneously published in the USA and Canada
by Routledge
711 Third Avenue, New York, NY 10017

Routledge is an imprint of the Taylor & Francis Group, an informa business

British Library Cataloguing in Publication Data
A catalogue record for this book is available from the British Library

Library of Congress Cataloging in Publication Data
Reed, Kate, 1972-
Gender and genetics : sociology of the prenatal / Kate Reed.
p. cm. – (Genetics and society)
Includes bibliographical references and index.
1. Genetic screening–Social aspects. 2. Ethnicity. I. Title.
RB155.65.R44 2012
362.196'04207–dc23
2011047966

ISBN: 978-0-415-55496-1 (hbk)
ISBN: 978-0-203-87002-0 (ebk)

Typeset in Times New Roman
by Taylor & Francis Books

For Ruby and Max

Contents

Acknowledgements x

Introduction 1

1 Information keeping/seeking 18

2 Gender, choice and time 39

3 Imaging and imagining genetics 59

4 Men, masculinity and decision-making 78

5 Gendering 'good' and 'bad' genes 96

6 Family, friends and heredity 115

7 Transforming social divisions 138

Conclusion 162

Appendix 181
Notes 183
Bibliography 185
Index 197

Acknowledgements

Many people helped with the production of this book. I would like first to thank the Wellcome Trust for funding the original project on which this book is based: 'Antenatal screening and the gendering of genetic responsibility'. Thanks also to all the male and female respondents who willingly contributed their time to be involved in the study. I would like to thank the midwives, screening specialists and other health professionals who made the study possible. I would also like to thank the midwives who participated in a related project on professional views about men's involvement. Special thanks go to Dr Kate Woodthorpe who conducted a number of interviews for the study along with a focus group interview with midwives. Thanks also go to my colleagues in the Department of Sociological Studies, University of Sheffield for their support, especially Dr Suzie Molyneux-Hodgson who is probably tired of listening to my endless discussions on genetics. Thanks also to other friends and medical professionals who advised me on the specifics of screening and scanning technologies and on genetically related fetal anomalies; particular thanks here go to Dr Elspeth Whitby Honorary Consultant Radiologist, University of Sheffield and Royal Hallamshire Hospital.

Thanks also go to friends and family. Thanks to Dr. Kirsten Macdonald for coffees, friendship and the wisdom of her medical knowledge and experience. Finally thanks to my family, my mum, dad and siblings. Particular thanks go to my two children Ruby and Max without whom the idea for this study/book would never have come to fruition, and of course to my wonderful husband Leo who as always makes everything possible.

Introduction

In 2005, during my first pregnancy I received a borderline positive screening result identifying me as a potential carrier for the inherited blood disorder beta thalassaemia. Under my local health care trust blood tests for thalassaemia were given universally to all women at around 12 weeks of pregnancy along with a whole battery of other tests ranging from my blood type to HIV testing. My partner and I were subsequently called back into the antenatal clinic where a genetic counsellor explained the implications of this screening result. Inherited blood conditions such as sickle cell anaemia and thalassaemia are conditions which mainly affect people who have originated from Africa, the Caribbean, the Middle East, Asia and the Mediterranean, but are also found in the northern European population. Inheritance of an affected gene from both parents leads to a 1 in 4 chance of the fetus developing either one of these disorders, whilst inheritance of one abnormal gene results in a healthy carrier (NHS Antenatal and Newborn Screening Programme 2008). Should a woman receive a positive test during prenatal screening for an inherited blood disorder, then their male partner will most likely also be offered blood screening.

The genetic counsellor in my case explained that we were 'low' risk because we were both ethnically white. However, in order to rule out the possibility of thalassaemia in the growing fetus, my husband was also asked to undergo screening. He was given a simple blood test similar to my own taken within the antenatal clinic. Alongside my husband, I was also retested to check my initial result. We sat together in the hospital antenatal clinic both tested at the same time. A midwife joked: 'This is fun, I don't normally get to stab men!' While I was pretty oblivious to the physical effects of blood tests, my husband had a less happy time. Much to his embarrassment he felt faint and nauseous after the blood was taken. He was advised to lie down on an examining table, and the midwives fetched him tea and biscuits. This caused some hilarity among the overwhelmingly female workforce in the unit. In the end my partner tested negative for the thalassaemia trait and therefore to his relief didn't require any further testing encounters. However, this whole experience, along with my broader observations of men's increasing involvement in the prenatal clinic piqued my interest in exploring gender roles in prenatal blood screening in more detail. In particular I wanted to explore both women and men's involvement – both genetic and social – during this process.

In 2006 therefore, I submitted a successful research proposal to the Wellcome Trust bioethics funding stream proposing a small qualitative study which focused on exploring gender roles and responsibilities in prenatal screening. The aim of this study was to explore men and women's roles and experiences of prenatal blood screening. The proposed study aimed to focus on blood screening for directly inherited disorders such as sickle cell anaemia and thalassaemia and serum screening for chromosomal anomalies such as Down's syndrome. My specific aims here were twofold: first, to focus on exploring gender roles when female partners underwent screening and second, if possible to include cases such as my own where men's genes also become subjected to scrutiny through male screening. The research proposal was successful and this book and several journal articles are the product of the research findings from the study (*see* Reed, 2009a, 2011a, 2011b).

The remainder of this introduction aims to examine existing debates on gender and prenatal screening along with providing information about the study on which the book is based. It will begin by exploring the gendered nature of reproduction and genetics, focusing on the differing roles ascribed to men and women in reproduction. It will move on to explore the cultural shifts in the ideology of fatherhood, highlighting the impact of men's increasing roles as fathers and supportive partners during pregnancy. The chapter will also explore existing literature on gender and screening, emphasising the neglect of men in existing research. As a theoretical underpinning for the rest of the book the chapter also offers a critical discussion of existing theories on gender roles and institutions. Furthermore, in order to provide a clear picture of prenatal screening, such as what tests are available, and what their results might mean for the pregnancy, the chapter will also give a detailed outline of the types of screening available to women throughout pregnancy in the UK. The introduction will move on to discuss the study itself. The aims, theoretical framework and methodology of the study will be outlined here, including a focus on such issues as sampling, data collection and analysis. The final section of the introduction will outline the book's structure, providing a brief synopsis of each chapter.

Gender, reproduction and genetics

Reproduction has formed the centre of much existing sociological and feminist research on women's health. Perhaps as a result studies on reproduction with a focus on gender tend to relate almost exclusively to women (Annandale and Clark 1996). As Delphy (1992) has pointed out, in existing literature the baby is invariably associated automatically with the woman who carried it. This, she argues, connects women's identity to motherhood and gives women greater rights over the baby than men. Sandelowski (1994) further articulates this connection. She argues that pregnant women have a privileged relationship to the fetus because they carry the fetus. Because women's knowledge of the fetus is embodied (a corporeal and concrete experience) they have a tactile awareness and sense of knowing the fetus that her men cannot share (Sandelowski 1994: 233–34). According to this viewpoint biological fatherhood, on the other hand, is a discontinuous experience; the genetic inseminator role is separated in time and space from the nurture role. Culturally and historically pregnancy and childbirth therefore has been and still are very largely the province of women (Meerabeau 1991). Women are portrayed as exclusive guardians of the fetus (Rapp 2000). In contrast men often appear to have limited or no roles in the process. Where they do, this is limited to that of genetic inseminator (Meerabeau 1991; Sandelowski 1994).

These differences in men and women's roles in reproduction can be directly mapped onto discussions of genetics. Scientific knowledge allocates each parent a 50 per cent contribution to the hereditary materials of a fetus during the moment of conception (Rapp 2000). However, in many cultures men are pictured as providing the creative seed or spark which causes the pregnancy without taking on any behavioural obligations which affect its outcome (Rapp 2000). Men appear to have a direct and positive 'blood' or genetic contribution through creating a life. Women's roles, on the other hand, are that of nurturer and fetal container (Ettorre 2002). It is up to women and their wombs to nurture men's genes to ensure they reach their full potential. Rothman (1986) locates these gender differences in patriarchal thought.[1] While the concept of patriarchy has had a variety of meanings, at its core is the recognition of paternity, the idea that children grow out of men's seeds. Through patriarchy a distinction is marked between 'seed' and 'soil' – between paternity and maternity (Rothman 1986). According to Rothman, men and their 'seed' are viewed as the potential, the 'life giver' the genetic connection. Women, on the other hand, represent the soil, the vessel for men's seed. According to Rothman (1995) this distinction is then upheld in the scientific field of genetics whereby genes and DNA are routinely associated with paternal ties whilst maternal ties continue to be associated with nurture and childrearing.

These gendered differences in reproduction and genetics have been further exacerbated with the emergence and development in reproductive technologies prevalent from the 1970s and 1980s onwards. These NRTs ranged from technologies such as abortion, through to IVF to prenatal genetic screening and diagnosis (Stanworth 1987). As these technologies emerged, several feminists warned of the patriarchal desire to control reproduction encased in such technological advances (Corea 1985). In this context feminists reinforced the importance of women's reproductive autonomy, emphasising the significance of women's rights to reproductive choice (Petchesky 1984). Over recent decades, however, many feminists have highlighted the potentially dual-edged nature of the quest for women's reproductive autonomy. Although autonomy offers choice for women, it also individualises reproductive decision-making, placing the enormity of responsibility in women's hands (Rapp 2000).

In light of this, studies have begun to challenge simplistic assumptions that the increasing use of genetic technology in pregnancy will inevitably lead to or reinforce patriarchal or male control (Markens, Browner and Preloran 2003). As highlighted in a number of studies, women are often the ones actively seeking out genetic technology, such as prenatal testing – they are not merely passive victims and pawns but active agents (Markens, Browner and Preloran 2003). Furthermore, men's roles cannot be reduced to that of genetic inseminators in reproduction as they are becoming increasingly socially involved fathers (LaRossa 1997). Therefore the gendered nature of genetics, reproduction and childbearing perhaps is more complicated than often presented in existing studies. The relationship between gender and genetics is something that the book aims to explore, with a specific focus on prenatal screening. In particular the book will explore the following questions: what roles do women and men take in prenatal screening? Do men take equal responsibility for the genetic health of the fetus? To what extent do women desire this involvement? In what ways do women see male involvement as an infringement on their reproductive autonomy? The book will focus on an exploration of gender as the social relations between the sexes (Reed 2006), with a focus on women and men's roles – both social and genetic – in prenatal screening.

Men, 'new fathers' and pregnancy

The expansion of men's roles in reproduction undoubtedly relates to a cultural shift in expectations surrounding fathering. This shift was most notable since the 1980s and driven in part by the very significant movement of mothers into the labour force (LaRossa 1988). Fathers in the 1950s–1970s have traditionally been presented as occupying distant, 'breadwinning', roles. In contrast the 'new father' of the 1980s and beyond has been perceived to be more emotionally involved, more nurturing and more committed to spending time with their children, during infancy and beyond (Wall and Arnold 2007). This has led some to suggest that we are moving towards the ideal of father as co-parent (Craig 2006).

The discourse of 'new fatherhood' signalled an expansion of men's roles not only in childrearing but also in their partners' pregnancies. As this discourse became established, research into men's experiences of their partners' pregnancies became more common both in the UK and US (e.g. Draper 2002, Jordan 1990). Recent reports by the World Health Organization (WHO 2007) have highlighted the important and mostly positive impact that men can have on their female partner's pregnancy and during the postpartum period. In a review of existing literature and research across Europe, the WHO (2007) concluded that during pregnancy and delivery, men can give important psychological and emotional support to women. This in turn can be shown to reduce pain, panic and exhaustion during delivery (Early 2001). Some studies have shown that men's presence in the labour room shortens the period of labour (Berry 1998). Some authors have even argued that men's nutritional interventions in pregnancy and labour has the potential to reduce the number of children born with low birth weight (Dudgeon and Inhorn 2004).

Due to the longstanding associations of pregnancy and childbirth with women, expectant fathers' experiences of their partners' pregnancies and their own transition to parenthood have not been nearly as well documented as those of motherhood. There are, however, several studies concerning expectant fathers' feelings, predominantly during the birth and the time afterwards (Barclay and Lupton 1999). For example, Finnbogadottir *et al.* (2003) conducted a Swedish study on the experiences of first time fathers. They found that first time fathers felt that they needed support and advice from health services during their partners' pregnancy. More recently, research has begun to explore the impact of pregnancy on men's mental and physical health (Bartlett 2004). Recent reports by the WHO (2007) have shown that increased involvement of men during pregnancy also benefits the man's health and wellbeing. For example, men who have been recognised in their new position as fathers and experienced emotional support during the pregnancy show better physical and mental health (Diemer 1997). The more the father engages himself during the birth and postnatal period the stronger the attachment to the baby (Sullivan 1999), and involvement as the child grows up (Chronholm 2004).

According to this stream of recent research, therefore, men's roles in pregnancy and childbirth have expanded considerably in a relatively short period of time. Men are no longer reduced to their biological role in conception but now take on a variety of social roles during pregnancy and beyond. Despite men's increasing involvement in childbearing and rearing however, some have urged caution. Some authors have pointed to a disconnection between the culture and practice of 'new fatherhood', with men widely being presented as more involved than they actually are in practice (LaRossa 1988). Subsequent research has certainly borne out the fact that although the conduct of fathers has changed, it is still mothers who bear the vast majority of responsibility for children (Craig 2006). Furthermore, as LaRossa (1997) pointed out, the cultural image of the 'new father' encourages men to be more active participants in childrearing. However, significant social and institutional barriers to greater father involvement still exist. According to Williams and Umberson (1999) these include gender roles that define men's role largely as breadwinner (Lorber 1994), workplace norms that discourage men from taking time off for children, and the relative lack of resources and institutional materials aimed at educating new and expectant fathers (Doyle 1995). In light of this, this book aims to explore gender roles in screening in the context of recent debates on fatherhood. In particular the book will explore the following issues: Does the practice of fatherhood mirror cultural shifts in the prenatal arena? To what extent do men and women continue to face ideological and institutional barriers towards men's greater participation? This is something which has so far received little attention in existing studies on prenatal screening.

Men, women and prenatal blood screening

Despite increasing academic interest in men's experiences of pregnancy, birth and fatherhood, there has been little research into men's experiences of their partners' prenatal screening and diagnosis (Green *et al.* 2004; Reed 2009a and 2011a). As with earlier research on pregnancy, most existing research on prenatal screening has tended to focus on women as the main recipients (Green *et al.* 2004). Where men's experiences in screening have been sought, these have tended to be in relation to their involvement in their partners' ultrasound scans. In particular, research has tended to highlight the benefits of ultrasound scans in enhancing men's experience of fatherhood during their partners' pregnancy.

In her UK-based study, for example, Draper (2002) notes the importance of ultrasound for helping men visualise the baby and realise their transition to fatherhood. In the US Sandeloswki (1994) highlights the ways that ultrasound makes parents' relationship to the fetus more equal, offering men access to a previously exclusively female world. In contrast to enhancing men's experiences of their partners' pregnancies, however, these studies have tended to highlight more of a mixed impact on women's experiences of imaging technology. When it comes the ways that ultrasound enables men to take a more equitable role in pregnancy Mitchell and Georges (1997) have argued that for women it offers the possibility of stimulating or engaging a partner's interest in the baby or testing their commitment to the relationship. At the same time while fetal ultrasound can enhance men's role in pregnancy it can also have the effect of minimising pregnant women's special relationship with the fetus whilst maximising their responsibility for fetal health and well-being (Sandelowski 1994).

However, while there are studies on men's involvement in ultrasound screening, their involvement in blood and serum screening is less well documented (Locock and Alexander 2006). Furthermore, men's experiences as recipients of screening are rarely explored (Reed 2009a, 2011). Whilst pregnant women are most likely to be the direct recipients of prenatal screening, as shown by the anecdote above men may also be screened for certain genetic disorders. Where both partners receive a positive test result for inherited blood disorders such as sickle cell and thalassaemia, women are offered further diagnostic testing (NHS Antenatal and Newborn Screening Programme 2008a). Despite men's potential involvement in this type of screening very few studies have included an analysis of gender roles in such screening (Chattopadhyay 2006).

This limited research on men's involvement in prenatal screening can be related to two issues already discussed: first, research focuses mostly on pregnant women because prenatal screening focuses mostly on the female body-mirroring those gendered associations of pregnancy and childbirth (Delphy 1992). Second, men are often reticent to take part in research on pregnancy and screening because it is perceived to be a women's issue (Rapp 2000).

However, as Sandelowski (1994) suggests, the importance and potential benefits and negative aspects of father involvement in screening continue to interest researchers (Jordan 1990). There is one recent study on serum screening and diagnostic testing which did include a focus on men's involvement in their partners' serum screening and diagnostic testing. This is Locock and Alexander's (2006) British study. Although this study focused primarily on women's experiences of prenatal screening it did also identify several potentially conflicting male roles in this process. Male roles identified in their study included: parents, a role often overlooked during women's prenatal screening; bystanders, men on the fringes of their partners' prenatal care; traditionally male roles of protectors/supporters; fact gatherers, involving practical info-gathering about screening; and finally decision-makers and enforcers. Locock and Alexander's (2006) study emphasises a need for further research on men's perceptions of prenatal screening. Building on some of the issues and themes raised by Locock and Alexander (2006), this book aims to explore both women and men's experiences and roles during screening. Before moving on to discuss the types of screening available in the UK and details of the study itself, I will give a brief outline of the theoretical framework to be used throughout the book.

Theoretical framework: Gendered roles and institutions

The aim of this book is to explore gender roles in prenatal screening with a focus on both women and men. Underpinning this exploration will be a focus on gender role ideology. The main focus of work on gender carried out during the 1970s and 1980s was on exploring the production of masculinity and femininity. Many feminist writers argued that gender is culturally determined and that we become differently gendered through socialisation into gender roles (Richardson 2008). Gender role ideologies are generally perceived as opinions and beliefs about the ways that private and public roles differ based on sex (Harris and Firestone 1998). Traditional roles are those that reinforce or conform to expected differences between men and women, whereas non-traditional roles depart from these expected differences (Harris and Firestone 1998). Traditional views on gender have placed the burden of pregnancy and child rearing on women and allocate men the traditionally masculine role of breadwinner (Lorber 1994; Lewis 2001). Recent research has focused on the ways in which there has been a move away from traditional gender roles in both private and public spheres to new and more complex forms of gender organisation (Scott 2006). Such shifts indicate the emergence of new forms of inequality and equality between men and women and among men and women themselves (Annandale and Hunt 2000).

Gender role ideology has been well criticised, not least because the approach tends to exaggerate the extent to which social life is scripted or prescribed (Annandale and Hunt 2000). For instance, there is often an underlying assumption that roles have the same meaning for men and women when they may actually have significantly different meanings for men and women in different social contexts (Clarke 1983). New conceptualisations of gender which were associated with the rise of postmodernism and queer theory emerging in the 1990s, shifted the emphasis away from definitions of gender as fixed coherent and stable, towards seeing gender categories as plural, provisional and situated (Richardson 2008). Subsequently recent research on gender focuses less on roles and more on the fluid and complex nature of subjectivity, diversity and the multiple constructions of femininity and masculinity (Francis 2008).

Despite its shortcomings, this book will draw on gender role ideology to explore gender roles in prenatal screening (see also Reed 2011a). As Markens, Browner and Preloran (2003) have shown although active agents, women (and men) continue to be constrained by the gendered institutions, roles and ideologies that shape their everyday lives and conditions of existence (Lorber and Bandlamudi 1993). Gender is an institution, a part of culture, a complex form of structured inequality (Lorber 1994). According to Ettorre (2002) it embeds into society a set of inter-related norms based on the activities of individuals and prescribes these activities. Thus individuals continue to be marked by differences on the basis of being male and female as well as masculine and feminine (Ettorre 2002). Whilst recognising that gender roles are far from fixed, the book will explore the kinds of roles women and men take during screening. In doing so it aims to examine how these are structured according to institutions of gender. The book asks: in what ways do gender roles in this context reinforce traditional male and female roles, and in what ways do they signify a transformation of these roles. In the following sections an overview of the types of prenatal screening available in the UK will be given in order to provide background context to the study.

Prenatal screening in the UK

Prenatal screening is the search for fetal abnormalities such as congenital malformations, chromosomal disorders, neural tube defects and genetic conditions among the asymptomatic population of pregnant women (Ettorre 2002: 23). In recent decades, advances in prenatal technology have led to improvements in the methods of detection of fetal abnormalities (Leshin 2007: 1). Such developments in types of technology continue apace. As a result types of prenatal screening available to women in the UK change on a regular basis. It is also important to note that although the term 'genetic screening' is widely adopted in the context of prenatal screening, primary tests themselves are not always directly genetics-based (Pilnick 2004). Furthermore, tests are also used to detect or predict the risk of a number of conditions only a handful of which are directly genetic in origin. Technologies may be used on their own or collaboratively in order to provide a better prediction of risk of certain types of anomalies, highlighting the potential 'need' for further diagnostic testing. Prenatal screening therefore is a conflicted, evolving and often ambiguous process which does not necessarily provide clear answers for pregnant women and their partners. It is however a key part of routine prenatal care in the UK. There are currently a number of screening and diagnostic tests available within the UK (although regional variation in what is and isn't offered free on the National Health Service (NHS) across the UK does exist). At the time of writing, the tests listed below were some of the key tests offered to women throughout the UK.

Screening for inherited conditions

Within the UK, in the first and second trimester of pregnancy women are offered a range of blood tests which include screening for maternal health and diseases (e.g. blood type, sexually transmitted diseases), and screening for fetal health. The latter tests include haemoglobinopathy screening for the sickle cell or thalassaemia trait. Sickle cell disorders (SCDs) and thalassaemia major are recessive conditions where individuals who inherit a deleterious gene from both parents develop the disease (Atkin, Ahmad and Anionwu 1998). These disorders are serious conditions. They affect the haemoglobin, a part of the blood that carries oxygen around the body. People who have these conditions will need specialist care throughout their lives (NHS Antenatal and Newborn Screening Programmes 2010).

As mentioned earlier, in the UK the groups more at risk are of African Caribbean descent and West African origin: thalassaemia is more common among Cypriots, South Asians and Chinese, but also occurs among white British and African-Caribbean people (Atkin, Ahmad and Anionwu 1998). Inheritance of an affected gene from both parents leads to a one in four chance of the fetus developing either one of these disorders, whilst inheritance of one abnormal gene results in a healthy carrier (NHS Antenatal and Newborn Screening Programme 2008). Under current NHS policy all women are offered a screening test for thalassaemia, however not all women will be offered a screening test for sickle cell. Whether a woman is offered sickle cell screening may depend on ethnicity and family history of both partners. A questionnaire is often used to identify those who are deemed at risk (NHS Antenatal and Newborn Screening Programmes 2010). If women test positive for the sickle cell or thalassaemia trait, however, then their male partners are also offered screening. If both partners are carriers couples are offered further diagnostic testing in order to determine whether a baby has either disorder (NHS Antenatal and Newborn Screening Programmes 2010).

Screening for chromosomal anomalies

Within the UK all women are universally offered screening tests for Down's syndrome although the specific type of test offered may vary across different health trusts. Down's syndrome is a condition which affects individuals to varying degrees. It tends to be associated with learning difficulties along with some health problems such as heart problems, reduced vision and hearing (NHS Antenatal and Newborn Screening Programmes 2011a). Down's syndrome is a chromosomal anomaly resulting from the production of a duplicate copy of chromosome 21 (also known as trisomy 21). Unlike blood disorders such as sickle cell and thalassaemia Down's syndrome is not a directly inherited condition.[2] In order to screen for Down's syndrome and other related conditions women are offered blood screening. Serum screening is carried out through a blood test to measure maternal serum alphafetoprotein (MSAFP) concentration. MSAFP levels may be combined with two other hormonal measures, estriol, and beta-hCG to produce what is called the 'triple test'. This test is usually conducted around 16 weeks of pregnancy and can then be used to estimate the risk of Down's syndrome. Although most commonly associated with screening for Down's syndrome, this blood screening can also be used to determine risks for other chromosomal anomalies such as Edward's and Turner's syndrome and neural tube defects such as spina bifida (Pilnick 2002).

During the last decade particular attempts have been made to improve screening for fetuses with chromosomal anomalies particularly Down's syndrome (Getz and Kirkengen 2003). A variety of combined blood and ultrasound tests are becoming increasingly available for this purpose. Tests offered in the UK include the combined and integrated tests. Nuchal fold (or nuchal translucency) scans form the centre of this type of screening. Nuchal scans measure the fluid between the neck, skin and spine. In fetuses affected by Down's syndrome, the nuchal fold tends to be thicker than in babies without Down's syndrome (Pilnick 2002). Recently nasal bone measurement has also been factored into this risk assessment for babies with Down's syndrome (NHS Evidence 2001). Despite advances in this type of screening, visual technologies such as ultrasound scans are not diagnostic, offering only an informed prediction of risk for chromosomal disorders. Depending on history and a calculation of risk assessment using these particular tests women may also be offered further diagnostic testing such as an amniocentesis (Pilnick 2002).

Fetal imaging: ultrasound and MRI

In the UK, a first visit to antenatal clinic often includes a trans-abdominal ultrasound often known as the 'dating' scan. This scan is used to confirm three things: that it is a viable pregnancy, that it is a single pregnancy and that the gestational age of the baby has been correctly estimated. Women are also offered a further routine ultrasound scan at around 20 weeks. During the scan, heartbeat and movement can be seen. This examination can also be used to exclude certain serious abnormalities, such as hydrocephalus, spina bifida, heart defects and kidney and bowel abnormalities. As with all antenatal procedures, not all abnormalities can be excluded on the basis of this scan (Pilnick 2002).

In recent years and as a result of refinement in technologies, clinical training and expertise, disclosure of more subtle structural abnormalities such as cleft palate is often possible through fetal ultrasound (Getz and Kirkengen 2003: 2046). Furthermore, since 1983 we have witnessed the emergence of fetal MRI (Magnetic Resonance Imaging) (Smith *et al.* 1983). This imaging technology can offer additional information not available by routine ultrasound so is consequently used when there is a suspected abnormality on the 20-week ultrasound scan. MRI is also used in cases where there is a strong family history of congenital abnormalities. It provides information on development of the brain that is not possible using ultrasound so gives additional information used to counsel the parents (Whitby *et al.* 2004). MRI is also useful when there are abnormalities in other body systems, for example the lungs or kidneys, although this is a new use and has not yet become well established.

Diagnostic testing

Diagnostic tests can be used to confirm the existence of a range of genetic and chromosomal anomalies in the fetus. It is often most commonly associated with the confirmation of Down's syndrome in a developing fetus. Two different types of diagnostic test are commonly used in the UK: chorionic villus sampling and amniocentesis. Chorionic villus can be carried out from around week 11 of pregnancy and involves a small needle being inserted through the abdomen under local anaesthetic and into the womb with the help of ultrasound. A small piece of placenta is then withdrawn and sent for testing. The test confirms the presence or absence of Down's syndrome by identifying abnormal chromosomes. However, the disadvantage of the test is that it can bring on a miscarriage in about 1 in a 100 women, regardless of whether or not any anomalies are found. Amniocentesis is also an invasive test: a small amount of the amniotic fluid is withdrawn using a needle around 16–18 weeks of pregnancy. The fetal cells are cultured and chromosomal abnormalities can be identified. This test is thought to carry a higher risk of miscarriage, approximately 1 in 50 (although this varies according to timing); the risk applies whether or not the fetus is identified with anomalies (Pilnick 2002: 64).

Gender and prenatal screening: The study

The research project on which this book is based focused on exploring gender roles and responsibilities within prenatal screening. As argued earlier, the study focused specifically on an analysis of blood screening for inherited blood disorders and chromosomal anomalies. However, as can be seen from the available screening technologies listed above, it is not always possible or appropriate to separate different types of tests. Furthermore, although the book focuses in particular on screening for inherited blood conditions and chromosomal anomalies, occasionally other genetic conditions were highlighted by respondents through their experiences of screening. Therefore, while focusing on particular types of screening and particular genetic and chromosomal disorders, the book draws on the respondents' accounts surrounding other technologies/conditions where appropriate. Furthermore, this book is focused on a study exploring the accounts of pregnant women and their partners. Subsequent data were also collected with health screening professionals such as midwives in order to obtain professional views on men's roles. However, these data are not included within this context here but is explored elsewhere in detail in other publications (Reed 2009b, 2011b).

Sampling and recruitment

This study took place in a northern city in the UK. Pregnant women were recruited to the study on receipt of NHS ethical approval and research governance from the relevant Local Research Ethics Committee and health authority.[3] Respondents were recruited and data collection commenced in late 2006. Twenty-two pregnant women and 16 of their male partners were recruited to the study, making 38 respondents in total (Reed 2009a, 2011a, 2011b). Despite the best efforts of both researchers fewer men than women were recruited to the study. As others have pointed out, men remain difficult to access in the women-centred antenatal realm (Rapp 2000).

Pregnant women were recruited through local NHS community and hospital midwives. Male partners were mostly recruited during their attendance to women's screening appointments. However, as men do not always attend routine prenatal appointments, they were also recruited through pregnant partners. There are drawbacks to recruiting men through their partners. As noted elsewhere, this could result in a self-selecting sample (Reed 2009a, 2011a). However, it is hoped that by adopting two different sampling strategies regarding male recruitment bias would be minimised. In order to adequately explore the screening process, pregnant female respondents were all at least 17 weeks' pregnant. To access a wide range of views on screening, respondents included women and men who were experiencing first, second and third, fourth and in one case fifth pregnancies. Within the study respondents were either married or unmarried but co-habiting. Respondents' ages ranged from 18 to 40. The study sought respondents who had received both high risk and normal screening results in order to access a range of screening experiences. It is important to note however that although several respondents received high-risk screening results and went on to have further screening and diagnostic testing, none of the respondents were diagnosed with inherited blood disorders or chromosomal anomalies. Therefore this study can make no comment on those who enter the realm of selective abortion (Reed 2009a, 2011a, 2011b).

Along with differences in age, number of pregnancies and screening results, different socio-economic groupings were also represented in the study.

Respondents included women and men from a range of occupations, the unemployed and those currently not looking for employment.[4] Some differences were less well represented in the study. For example, the majority of respondents were ethnically white. Two respondents identified as Black African, three as South Asian, one as Mauritian,[5] one as Czech two as white Irish and the rest as white British. As argued by many researchers it is often difficult to recruit women of colour and working class women in research on pregnant women and prenatal care (Lazarus 1994, Rowe and Garcia 2003). However, as Earle and Letherby (2007) have pointed out, it is difficult to represent the experiences of everyone in research. A summary of all female and male respondents interviewed as part of this study can be found in the appendix of this book.[6]

Data collection and analysis

The study took an *inductive* approach to data collection (Bryman 2001). Therefore it did not begin with a hypothesis but rather set out to empirically explore a general set of research problems (Bryman 2001). From the outset several research problems were identified: does gender influence choice and decision-making in prenatal screening and, if so, in what ways does it do so? What roles do women and men take throughout screening? Does gender affect potential parental feelings of genetic responsibility? If so, how does this affect decisions made about screening and diagnostic testing? In what ways do the roles that men and women take during screening reflect or challenge traditional gender roles (Reed 2007b, 2009a, 2011a, 2011b)?

In order to empirically address these research problems a method was needed which generated 'open' data rather then imposing a formalised set of questions (Oakley 1981). Semi-structured interviewing was selected for this purpose. The interview schedule was based around screening procedures themselves and the decision-making process. Examples of the types of interview questions asked included: which blood tests are opted for and why? Do couples decide which tests to opt for together or does one partner take a more active role in making decisions about screening? Do men and women make decisions about diagnostic tests as a couple or does one partner take more responsibility? Data were collected between January 2007 and August 2007. Interviews were conducted by the primary investigator and one researcher through the use of an agreed interview schedule. Interviews were conducted in prenatal clinics and in people's homes or in a location suitable to them.

In total 32 interviews were conducted. In order to maximise participation respondents were given the option of being interviewed together or individually. Twelve respondents were interviewed as couples and the rest were interviewed separately. It is acknowledged that this approach might lead to the production of different types of data. As Hirsch (1993) argues in his study on IVF, interviewing couples together can place limits on topics discussed as individuals may feel inhibited by one another's presence. Throughout this study on prenatal screening, there seemed to be no obvious differences in the nature of topics discussed between couple or individual interviews. In fact utilising the two types of interview appeared to enhance the production of data. It enabled the interviewer's access to the rich dynamics of couple's interactions as well as providing contrasts to individual interviews (Markens, Browner and Preloran 2003). In order to ensure consistency between interviews, however the same interview schedule was used throughout.

The majority of interviews took place on a face-to-face basis. However, due to time constraints two of the male respondents were interviewed by telephone. Bryman (2001) has pointed to the potential pitfalls of using telephone interview, for example, the inability of the interviewer to draw on observation as a prompt in the interview process. During this study however, the telephone interviews captured some interesting and detailed data. All interviews were tape recorded and lasted approximately one hour. In order to ensure confidentiality of respondents all their names have been changed and transcripts made anonymous. The data were transcribed and analysed thematically. The process of data analysis took several stages. Initially transcripts were coded and organised into themes and categories. The identified themes included: reproductive choice, reproductive gate-keeping, decision-making, diagnostic testing, genetic responsibility, gender roles in pregnancy and screening, male involvement, interactions with health professionals, family and peer groups. Social theories about the gender roles and responsibilities in screening were then developed from these themes. This book is based explicitly on data collected during the study. These data may at times appear contradictory as respondents sometimes articulated a paradoxical set of views. However, the aim of this book has been to adhere as faithfully as possible to original accounts. In the final section of this chapter I will outline the structure and content of the rest of the book.

Structure of the book

The book is divided into seven substantive chapters in total. Chapter 1 focuses on exploring gender roles around information sought/disseminated about prenatal screening. It will begin with a focus on the ways in which women establish their roles as guardians of fetal health through gate-keeping information about genetic screening. Women seek out information about pregnancy and genetic screening and selectively disseminate that information to partners, thus reinforcing their role as guardians of the fetus. This role is further supported by midwives and other health professionals who disseminate screening information only to women. As the chapter will move on to explore however, this female exclusivity in the realm of prenatal genetics is currently being challenged by an increase in men's access to information about genetic screening (Locock and Alexander 2006), particularly through men's use of information technology. As argued elsewhere, the Internet constitutes a unique medium where 'expert' knowledge on health is accessible to anyone with a networked computer (Hardey 1999). Men use the Internet to seek out information on pregnancy, screening and genetic conditions. This allows them access to a previously exclusive female world, thus challenging women's roles as exclusive guardians of fetal health.

Concepts of choice and time form the centre of Chapter 2. These concepts have been fundamental to debates on both the new genetics and human reproduction. For example, some social theorists have placed the new genetics firmly in the domain of individual choice (Rose 2001). More cynical authors however point to the increasing routinisation of technology (Kerr 2004), particularly with regard to prenatal screening (Press and Browner 1997). The concept of time has also been central to debates on reproductive technology (Earle and Letherby 2007). Women's reproductive bodies are constrained by time and as Grosz (1999) argues, women are granted no time or space of their own. As will be articulated within this chapter, time and choice are crucial to an analysis of gender and genetic screening. Drawing on data from the study this chapter will explore the intersections between gender, choice and time. Throughout screening women and men make choices about which tests to opt for. These choices are routinised and placed in a set of temporal constraints. Women are constrained by their own corporeality as screening for genetic conditions and chromosomal anomalies must take place during certain periods of gestation. Men are constrained by social and institutional barriers, for example, workplace norms that discourage them from taking time off to participate in screening (Williams and Umberson 1999). The chapter will conclude by questioning the notion of 'choice' in screening, highlighting the ways in which choices made about screening are mediated and constrained by gender, time and materiality.

Chapter 3 focuses on an exploration of gender dynamics in relation to different types of reproductive technology. Drawing on empirical data from the study, this chapter will focus on the distinctions made by men and women between blood screening and visual screening such as ultrasound scanning. Within this study both women and men distinguished between genetic blood screening and ultrasound scans. Both saw the scans as more important in detecting genetic conditions and fetal anomalies because they gave visual evidence of the health of the fetus. A particular set of gender roles were then mapped onto these distinctions. Women and their DNA were associated with serum screening, men and their genes were associated with ultrasound. This chapter will explore these differences in order to emphasise the importance of 'visual markers' in enabling men to connect with their offspring (Sandelowski 1994), reaffirming also women's secondary role in genetic progress as fetal containers (Ettorre 2000).

Much existing research on prenatal screening focuses on pregnant women as the moral guardians of decision-making. Women make decisions over which tests to opt for, and what to do if prenatal screening and diagnostic results are positive (Rothman 1986). While partners, the medical profession and family are given some consideration in existing research on decision-making, the 'totality' of the maternal role as the source of the gravity with which decisions are made is emphasised (Ivry 2007: 253). Drawing on data from the study, Chapter 4 will highlight the importance of men's roles in decision-making, situating these roles in broader debates on 'the new fatherhood' (La Rossa 1997). As the data will show, men often take key roles in decision-making, both with regard to chromosomal anomalies such as Down's syndrome and screening for inherited blood disorders. This is despite pressure from health professionals for women to take the key role in decision-making. The chapter will move on to explore the implications of this increase in men's roles as decision-makers. Does it emphasise a shift towards more equal gender roles and responsibilities in screening or does it merely signify an extension of male control over women in reproduction?

In existing literature on reproduction, men have often been associated with the production of so called 'good genes'. Men seeds and semen are viewed as the 'sparks', the 'life givers' of pregnancy while women are arguably perceived as caretakers of the fetus (Rothman 1986). However, should women receive positive prenatal screening results or diagnosis then they are often viewed by society as bad reproducers, with ineffective wombs accused of producing children with faulty genes (Finger 1990; Ettorre 2000). Drawing on data from the study, this chapter will explore the gendered association of so-called 'good' and 'bad' genes in prenatal screening. As the findings of the study show, men are often concerned with the establishment of routine genetic (blood) connections between themselves and the fetus while women often take responsibility for positive or 'high-risk' screening results. However, the chapter will move on to show that maternal responsibility for the production of faulty genes is not straightforward but is complexly mediated by a number of other factors including ethnicity and screening type (Reed 2009a). Furthermore, men do take responsibility for the production of 'bad' genes in screening, particularly when they too have to be screened – as may be the case in screening for inherited blood disorders. Thus as will be argued, the gendering of good and bad genes is complex and contradictory, both challenging and reinforcing a traditional set of gender roles.

Chapter 6 aims to situate the gendered nature of prenatal screening in a broader social context. It will explore the importance of external factors such as family and friends on gender dynamics in prenatal screening. The chapter will begin with an exploration on the influence of friends. Throughout the study friends often influenced couples' decisions to opt for certain types of prenatal screening – particularly the use of privately funded technology such as Nuchal Fold screening. Family also strongly affected screening decisions and often contributed to conflicts between men and women. Family influence in screening also has a more direct influence on genetics and gender roles (Rapp 2000). As will be explored, within the study respondents often had a general awareness of the role of family genetic history. At times this awareness of history affected attitudes towards prenatal screening – particularly in cases where family members suffered from various inherited disorders. Family history also had direct clinical implications when genetic links were identified, sought out and monitored. Overall then the chapter will emphasise the positive roles that family and friends can play in couples' experiences of prenatal screening – both indirectly through supporting women and their partners during screening and more directly through family history and inheritance. However, the chapter will also emphasise the ways in which family and friends also lead to gendered conflicts between couples – and again tends to reinforce the gendered nature of genetic responsibility.

The final substantive chapter takes a much broader comparative approach to the examination of gender and prenatal genetics. The aim of this final substantive chapter is to explore the potential of new technologies such as prenatal screening techniques to transform existing social relationships more broadly. In this context it will move away from focusing its exploration explicitly on gender roles. It will focus instead on the relationships between prenatal screening and other types of social stratification including social class and race and ethnicity. Drawing on data from the study, along with a wider body of literature on inequality and screening, this chapter will argue that technologies such as prenatal screening do present some challenges to existing forms of inequality. As will be shown, through the data, while some social divisions existed between respondents along the lines of social class and race and ethnicity (e.g. access to certain types of technology) these should not be overestimated. Women and men's roles in prenatal screening in this study both challenged and reflected existing forms of stratification – including class, race and gender. The chapter will conclude by evaluating the role of technology itself in transforming social relationships. It will conclude by examining the role of prenatal screening technology itself in either transforming or reinforcing existing social circumstances?

The final chapter of the book will conclude by arguing that the gendered nature of screening is paradoxical. Rapp (2000) argues that screening acts as a forum for the making and re-making of gender roles. According to her screening marks the start of a traditionally gendered set of parenting roles. However, as argued throughout the book, the gendered nature of prenatal screening is more complicated than often thought. The structured process of prenatal screening does seem to foster traditional views on pregnancy. However, it is also a platform which illustrates gender change as men become more active participants in pregnancy and screening – including taking responsibility for their own genetic input into the health of the fetus. As will be explored, these changes are indicative of the nature of gender roles in contemporary British society more generally – as existing gender roles continue to be publicly and privately both reinforced and challenged (Reed 2006). The book will conclude by arguing for the need to give greater consideration to men's roles in screening, focusing on the implications of this for future research and practice.

1 Information keeping/seeking

Introduction

Existing studies have shown that throughout pregnancy women seek out and are targeted with a range of information on pregnancy and screening. Such information ranges from formal information disseminated by health professionals orally or through leaflets, books, etc., to informal sources of information textbooks/magazines/pregnancy support groups (Marteau and Dormandy 2001; Lowe *et al.* 2009). While many authors have highlighted the benefits of women seeking/receiving such information (Marteau and Dormandy 2001), others have been more scathing, viewing this information as yet another form of biomedical regulation of women's bodies (Marshall and Woollett 2000). One issue that is apparent however in existing research is that women remain the key targets/recipients of pregnancy-related information, emphasising their roles as exclusive guardians of fetal and child health (Rapp 2000). Little is known about men's involvement in this process of information seeking (Locock and Alexander 2006). The aim of this chapter is to explore both women and men's roles as information seekers, disseminators and consumers focusing on the ways in which this has the potential to both reinforce and challenge a traditional gender division of labour in reproduction.

Drawing on data from the study, the first two sections of the chapter will focus on women's roles as key targets, seekers and consumers of pregnancy-related information. Women seek out information about pregnancy and genetic screening and selectively disseminate that information to partners, thus reinforcing their role as guardians of the fetus. As will be argued women establish their roles as guardians of fetal health through gate-keeping information about genetic screening. Traditional gender roles in reproduction are therefore reinforced with women taking more responsibility for the health of the fetus. This role is further supported by midwives and other health professionals who disseminate screening information predominantly to women. As the chapter will move on to explore however, this female exclusivity in the realm of prenatal genetics is currently being challenged by an increase in men's access to information about genetic screening (Locock and Alexander 2006), particularly through men's use of information technology. As argued elsewhere, the Internet constitutes a unique medium where 'expert' knowledge on health is accessible to anyone with a networked computer (Hardey 1999). Men use the Internet to seek out information on pregnancy, screening and genetic conditions. This allows them access to a previously exclusive female-only world, thus perhaps challenging women's roles as exclusive guardians of fetal health. The chapter will conclude therefore by emphasising the 'gender paradox' surrounding women and men's roles around information seeking/receiving, on the one they hand signal a reinforcement of traditional gender roles whilst attempting to move beyond them on the other.

Women, information and pregnancy

According to Lowe *et al.* (2009) as far as we can tell, women have always sought out and been given advice about pregnancy, although the sources of information have varied over time. In the UK information is presented using one or more media, most often orally and in writing by health care professionals providing prenatal care. In recent years there has also been an increase in dissemination of pregnancy information on the web (Marteau and Dormandy 2001). In the UK sources of information have ranged from official texts such as *The Pregnancy Book* (DoH 2006) and *Emma's Diary* (Royal College of General Practitioners 2005) to leaflets produced by primary care or hospital trusts. There is also a range of books and magazines offering advice and guidance such as *Pregnancy and Birth Magazine* or self-help books such as *What to Expect When You're Expecting* (Murkoff and Mazel 2009). In addition to printed sources, women also share pregnancy and birth stories with other women through various antenatal leisure groups for example, pregnancy yoga, prenatal swimming or National Childbirth Trust (NCT 2011) classes. Consequently seeking and receiving different forms of information could be considered a normal part of pregnancy (Lowe *et al.* 2009).

Along with printed sources of information, oral advice given by midwives is one of the most important ways of disseminating information on antenatal care to pregnant women (Marteau and Dormandy 2001). Much of the discourse surrounding information disseminated by midwives (certainly when it comes to screening) focuses on enabling women to make informed choices about whether or not to opt for particular tests. According to guidelines by NICE (2003b) women and their partners should be informed of tests. Midwives are encouraged to highlight the use of such tests in enabling the best possible care is provided for women during pregnancy whilst also emphasising the importance of individual choice (see Chapter 2). The UK screening commission emphasises the importance of midwives engaging in annual revision/updating sessions on developments in genetic testing in order that they are able to give women the best possible advice (UK Screening Committee 2003).

Studies have shown that women value high-quality information given personally by health professionals and as early as possible in prenatal care to allow for reflection and informed decision-making (Carroll *et al.* 2000,

Marteau and Dormandy 2001). However, despite women's desire for good-quality information, recent studies in both the US and UK have highlighted significant variation in the quality of information available. Studies in the UK analysing written information have often judged these to be poor quality in terms of factual information covered (Murray *et al.* 2001). According to Marteau and Dormandy (2001) oral information has often shown to have more of an impact on women than written information. However, women are also critical of this type of information often deeming it to be misleading and insufficient. For example, health professionals disseminating screening information may not know about certain conditions found in pregnancy and fetal health, may not have adequate counselling skills, or may simply not have time to go through things thoroughly. Therefore existing studies show that while important, pregnancy information disseminated to women can be of varying quality.

A number of feminist authors have further queried the dissemination and content of information given to pregnant women, arguing that it is part of a further medical regulation of women and their bodies. Marshall and Woollett (2000) for example analysed a number of pregnancy texts/guides. They argue that a number of disciplinary practices are at work in such texts both in planning for pregnancy and through making women responsible for fetal health during pregnancy. Pregnancy texts encourage women to take on board healthy lifestyles which reinforce the importance of contact with health professionals, emphasising a repertoire of pregnancy at risk (Marshall and Woollett 2000). According to them, such practices serve to mask diversity and to decontextualise and individualise pregnancy. This then separates pregnancy from women's other relationships, identities and knowledges with little regard to the circumstances in which women become pregnant (Marshall and Woollett 2000). This critique highlights an important issue to be explored in the context of this chapter – that is that traditional forms of pregnancy information are aimed at women. They emphasise the importance of women and maternal responsibility in pregnancy thus reinforcing women's central roles as mothers and as guardians of fetal health (Rapp 2000).

Some of the problems raised by traditional forms of pregnancy information dissemination have perhaps been addressed through women's use of the Internet. The Internet has great potential in pregnancy for providing tailored information to meet women's needs. A number of authors have already emphasised the Internet as a great resource for women during pregnancy. For example, Lowe *et al.* (2009) in their secondary analysis of interview data with pregnant women and their partners found that the Internet was a particular useful resource for women when experiencing problematic pregnancy ('problematic' is used to describe women's understanding that their pregnancy is problematic in some biological way). Lowe *et al.* (2009) found that often when a problematic pregnancy was defined, women had to look for information sources that went beyond their traditional ones and this is where the Internet was particularly useful. Recent studies have also shown that the Internet can be useful in increasing men's roles in pregnancy and screening. In their study Locock and Alexander (2006) found that one of the roles men took during their pregnant partners' screening was that of 'gatherer and guardian of fact'. Within their study men sought out information about testing available and about the types of conditions found through screening. The findings of their study show that one of the issues that have increased men's roles in this context is the Internet. Within their study there were accounts of men spending time searching the Internet and taking the lead in asking questions during consultations with health professionals. This is something that will be explored in greater detail in this chapter.

This chapter will explore gender roles in pregnancy information seeking, consuming and disseminating in relation to prenatal blood screening. Most of the chapter will focus on exploring routine screening and 'normal' screening results; however, where possible the chapter includes an exploration on information seeking when women are experiencing potentially problematic pregnancies. The chapter will first explore traditional types of information given to women in pregnancy, focusing on analysing the importance of such information to women during pregnancy. The chapter will move on to explore the gendered nature of information seeking. It will highlight the ways in which women actively seek out information about pregnancy and screening, taking the major role in disseminating it to male partners and encouraging partners to read such information. In doing so the chapter makes the argument that information seeking/consuming by both men and women reinforces women's roles as guardians and gatekeepers of pregnancy. The role of health professionals will also be explored here. In particular, the chapter will focus on the ways in which the roles of health professionals tend to facilitate women's position as guardians of fetal health. The final section of the chapter will move on to explore the ways in which these roles are perhaps shifting through men's increased use of the Internet to seek out pregnancy-related information.

Women as information seekers and recipients

In support of the findings of earlier studies, most women within the study discussed the ways in which they sought out and used pregnancy-related information. Women relied on information disseminated from a range of traditional sources such as oral information and leaflets given during routine antenatal care by midwives. Women also sought out other non-traditional sources such as the Internet as can be seen in the account from Liz who was in the third trimester of pregnancy:

> I actively found stuff out you know, about the tests and that. You know, I read the leaflets that the midwife gave me and I went on the net to look around, especially about the Down's testing. What it meant. What the chances were and that.
>
> (Liz, 32, University researcher)

Again, as with existing research on pregnancy, many women within this study wanted to receive information early on so they could make informed choices about the various tests available. Women tended to view this positively as highlighted by Katarina who was at the end of her first trimester of pregnancy with twins:

> Actually, again like you say, I just want to know everything as early as possible, at the earliest possible point, then you can make a decision one way or the other, and then you can get used to that then.
>
> (Katarina, 28, Self-employed)

Some women found the amount of information that they received was overwhelming. In fact some women didn't read everything as they felt that there was just too much information. This can be seen in the account from Rosie who was in the second trimester of her fifth pregnancy:

> Well, they did give us lots of information, in fact I were a bit overwhelmed by it, endless leaflets and stuff. Also, there was loads of stuff in the bounty pack (free information pack given to women at the start of pregnancy) about pregnancy and testing. I never really got chance to read them and that.
>
> (Rosie, 28, Housewife)

Women sometimes felt that the information given to them during routine antenatal clinic was repetitive. This can be seen in the account from Chelsea who was in the third trimester of pregnancy:

> I did read everything that the midwives gave us you know about the tests but I have to say a lot of it was very repetitive. I actually found that talking to my friends was the best thing, you know, the ones that had already gone through pregnancy.
>
> (Chelsea, 25, Care-worker)

Other women felt that the information they received during antenatal clinic on issues relating to screening was quite limited in terms of content. This can be seen in the quote from Emily who was in the second trimester of pregnancy:

> Erm, I think it's quite limited, the role that the hospital was playing, I don't think they inform you that much about it, about the choices you can make. But maybe that was because they assumed that I would know anyway, because I do feel quite confident in the choices that I make, so they don't ask the questions, so maybe that's why we don't have those discussions.
>
> (Emily, 30, Health professional)

Some women felt that the formal information disseminated by health professionals in the hospital could be quite intimidating. Again in support of earlier studies women found that the information they got through other women and pregnancy groups was more useful and reassuring (the role of friends will also be explored in more detail in Chapter 6). This can be seen in the account from Katarina who was at the end of her first trimester of pregnancy with twins:

KATARINA: The hospital information is great but a bit frightening, pregnancy twin group is better especially the birth stories at the end (of the session), they take the fear away.

INTERVIEWER: Is that something that you do on a regular basis?

KATARINA: Yes, we meet once a week and swap stories about pregnancy and birth. It's really helpful, you know to hear other people's experiences and know that you're not alone, especially when you are having twins!

(Katarina, 28, Self-employed)

Women who were experiencing their second or third pregnancy generally seemed to feel that they were already more informed as this wasn't their first pregnancy. However, women who had been through the process already were sometimes still sceptical about the information they had received. Some women felt that midwives didn't give them enough information about the tests and just performed them without too much discussion. This was especially the case with the first set of blood tests as can be seen in the account from Suzie who was in the second trimester of pregnancy:

> Erm, I think I'm quite well informed. But I don't know whether that's because it's the second time, or not. I mean, you're sort of sat down in a room having a load of blood tests and that in your arm, but you don't particularly know why. And then the results come back and it's like everything's fine, and you sort of think, what have they tested for? You know, why? Why did they take all that blood? Why do this and that? And I don't know, you don't particularly get any information from the staff at the hospital, as to why they're doing all this.
>
> (Suzie, 34, Wages clerk)

Most women within the study discussed traditional forms of information seeking and dissemination although views on information seeking and the usefulness of information varied. In concurrence with earlier studies women often sought out a range of information about pregnancy and screening (Lowe *et al.* 2009). Sometimes women saw this information as beneficial sometimes they were more critical both of quantity and quality of the information given. They were often more critical of the dissemination of formal types of information, for example, from health professionals. Often women felt the best information was that given to them by other pregnant women.

Gender and screening information

Most existing studies on pregnancy that have included an analysis of the role of information seem to focus mostly on women. In some cases parents are referred to rather than either mothers or fathers; however, the focus is seldom on fathers in particular. This is unsurprising given that women are the ones experiencing pregnancy. Furthermore, as argued earlier, this also undoubtedly reflects the lack of research more generally on men's roles in pregnancy. However, as stated in the introduction recent studies in prenatal screening have begun to include a focus on men's roles. For example, in their study on screening and diagnostic testing Locock and Alexander (2006) identified a number of potentially conflicting male roles during screening and prenatal diagnosis. This ranged from men's roles as parents through to decision-makers and enforcers. One of the male roles identified in their study was that of 'gatherers' and 'guardians' of fact. Locock and Alexander (2006) found that one way for men to channel their anxiety and try to support their partner during screening and diagnosis of fetal anomaly was through practical information-gathering. Within their study there were accounts of men spending time searching the Internet and taking the lead in asking questions. Some women felt that they were more inclined to respond intuitively whilst their male partners wanted as much 'hard fact' as possible. Draper (2002) shows in her study on men and pregnancy that some men highlight the importance of the acquisitions of 'technical knowledge' on pregnancy, arguing that for some men this resonates with more traditional discourses on masculinity. In existing studies therefore, men took a key role in information seeking, a role that resonates with traditional forms masculinity (Connell 2000)

Drawing on the findings of this study, the aim of this section of the chapter is to explore gender roles around information, seeking, disseminating and consuming. As will be shown within this next section, when it came to traditional sources of information seeking (such as oral information and printed sources such as leaflets/books) women within this study took a more significant role in the process. Women acted as information seekers and disseminators reinforcing in the process their role as gatekeepers of fetal health. Men on the other hand seldom sought out information and were often reluctant consumers of pregnancy information.

Women seeking, men (reluctantly) reading

Female respondents talked at length about seeking, disseminating and consuming information with male partners. Overall women appeared to take the major role in seeking traditional sources of pregnancy-related information for example seeking oral and printed pregnancy-related information. Men rarely sought out these traditional sources of information and were mostly reluctant information consumers. Several women discussed the ways in which they read through leaflets together with their male partners as a couple and as potential parents. In talking about whether both men and women read leaflets, the response from Emma in the second trimester of pregnancy was quite common for information about routine screening: 'Yeah, we both read through them together' (Emma, 22, Nanny). One couple who had received 'risky' blood screening results talked about the ways in which they read printed information together as a couple. For example, Flo had received a high-risk result for Down's screening and subsequently went on to have an amniocentesis. She was given leaflets on this type of diagnostic testing and on the potential outcomes by her midwife. She was clear in her interview that this information had been read by both her and her partner Paul: 'The midwife turned up at the house with the results and Paul (Flo's partner) was there. She gave us loads of information about the amniocentesis and we sat and read it together' (Flo, 35, Self-employed).

However, while several women discussed the ways in which they read leaflets together with their male partners as a couple, women did tend to feel that they had done the majority of information seeking and disseminating. For example, again as Emma articulates she conducted all the information seeking about pregnancy and routine screening not her partner:

> I feel I have to be. Obviously he's read everything, but I've looked into things more, like on the Internet. Things like I haven't understood what kind of test and stuff, I've had a quick glance or I've asked my Mom, or someone else, and they've said oh it's such and such or whatever. But he's (male partner) only vaguely glanced upon it, but checked out what these tests are.
>
> (Emma, 22, Nanny)

It wasn't just a case of women seeking and men reading information however; many women felt that they engaged with information more fully than their male partners. This can be seen in the comments below from Zoe who was in the third trimester of pregnancy and her partner Dave:

INTERVIEWER: And did you get all the information, all the leaflets and things.
ZOE: Yes.
INTERVIEWER: Did you both read them?
ZOE: I read them! (both laugh).
DAVE: I did read the covers.
INTERVIEWER: Why was that?
DAVE: I just got the information I wanted out of them, didn't feel the need to read them.
ZOE: I think I was probably just reading everything about pregnancy to be honest!

(Zoe, 31, Museums officer and Dave, 31, Graphic designer)

Men were often very honest when it came to discussions about leaflets and written information. They often stated that they simply weren't as interested in it as their female partners were. This can be seen in the quote from Brendan whose partner Liz was in the third trimester of pregnancy: 'We got a little pack (of information), but there was nothing in there that you didn't know already. I won't say both of us (read it) because I haven't read as much' (Brendan, 33, Travel agent).

Some women felt that their male partners didn't take as much of an interest in leaflets and written information. However, women didn't always view this negatively as they often felt that information was more directly related to them than to their partners. This reinforces accounts in other studies that highlight the ways in which men think pregnancy and pregnancy-related issues are mostly meant just for women (Rapp 2000; Markens, Browner and Preloran 2003). It also reinforces a traditional gender division of labour when it came to roles and pregnancy and child rearing whereby women take the major responsibility for maintaining fetal health while men are estranged from the process. This can be seen in the account from Suzie who was in the second trimester of pregnancy:

INTERVIEWER: Did he ever read any of the information leaflets? I mean you read them?

SUZIE: Yes.

INTERVIEWER: And does he read them?

SUZIE: Not particularly as much as I would, because I would read them straight away. And I'd leave them and say, oh I've got from the doctors or whatever it was, and maybe he would go through it, but I think he actually thinks it concerns me, not him.

(Suzie, 34, Wages clerk)

Within the study some men distinguished between written information and oral information given by midwives. They felt that while they didn't bother with seeking out or reading written information such as leaflets they did listen to information given by midwives and they did ask questions. This can be seen in the account from Pete whose partner Rosie was having her fifth baby:

INTERVIEWER: And do you ever read any information you're given like NHS things?

PETE: Not really. Not unless something specific. If the midwife, I mean when the midwife's here I do try and ask questions if I don't understand, but again if I'm at work (it's difficult). The only time I've been at home when midwife's come round I've had an illness so I've been off (work). And I do try and talk, try and find out, and I'd like to know, I always like to know what the next stage (of pregnancy) is.

(Pete, 31, Plasterer)

There was one man in the study who seemed to actively seek out more information than his pregnant partner. This was William a doctor, who gathered information on various screening procedures, disseminated information to his partner Lucy who was in the second trimester of pregnancy. In fact, Lucy joked during the interview that he knew more about her pregnancy than she did.

WILLIAM: I wanted to find out as much as possible about screening, about what was available on the NHS and privately. I wanted to do as much as possible to help Lucy and share the burden.

LUCY: Actually. I think he knows more about pregnancy then me!

(William, 35, GP and Lucy, 35, Hospital doctor)

It appeared that when it came to information seeking, especially with regard to written information, women sought out and read information thoroughly. Men on the other hand were rarely involved in information seeking and were often even rather reluctant to consume written information such as that from printed sources. Men often waited for their partners to take the lead role in information seeking expecting women to disseminate information to them. As will be explored in the next section, this was often used by women to ensure their role as guardian of fetal health.

Women as information gatekeepers

Several women within the study felt information should be directed at them because they were the ones who were pregnant. As argued earlier, a more traditional set of gender roles in reproduction was then reinforced in this context. Women sought out and thoroughly engaged with material on pregnancy and screening whereas men took much more of a secondary role in the process. Women's accounts highlighted another of women's key roles in pregnancy as disseminators of information. Women often felt that men would not have taken any interest in information themselves had their female partners not passed information onto them in the first place. This can be seen in the account below from Emily in the second trimester of pregnancy.

> Yeah, erm, I think his role is different to mine; he doesn't read all the magazines and leaflets to the extent that I do. I think I get, fortunately I get a lot of pleasure out of being pregnant, and so I get right into it. For him, I think he's happy to hear about my enthusiasm about it, but I don't think I would ever see him pick up a leaflet and be sat there thinking about the risks or something. If I hadn't given it him and discussed it with him he wouldn't go out of his way to find out.
>
> (Emily, 30, Health professional)

Male respondents also discussed women's roles as disseminators of pregnancy information. This can be seen in the account from Dave whose partner Zoe was in the third trimester of pregnancy: 'Zoe probably read more of the background information. Everything that Zoe read she passed on to me; it kind of worked out that way' (Dave, 31, Graphic designer). In many cases women saw themselves as disseminators and gatekeepers of pregnancy information. They decided what and how much information about pregnancy and screening was meted out to their male partners. This can be seen in the account from Suzie, who was in the second trimester of pregnancy:

SUZIE: I think so, yeah. Maybe because I told him we're going for a scan and having that blood test.

INTERVIEWER: So you were the information keeper.

SUZIE: (laughs) Yeah.

INTERVIEWER: And sort of telling him what's going on.

SUZIE: Yeah, yeah. Which is only natural because I'm getting the letters with the dates on and where to go, what's going to happen, and I tell him, so yeah.

INTERVIEWER: Would it help if letters were addressed to him in that way?

SUZIE: No I don't think it would. Maybe it would, you know, he'd be a bit more informed, but I'm a bit of a control freak. I like to have my name on the letter and it telling *me* what to do. And then I tell him.

(Suzie, 34, Wages clerk)

Although women wanted men to be involved and share in pregnancy and screening information, they wanted to be the ones who had ultimate control. They wanted to decide how much men knew about pregnancy-related issues. This then emphasises women's roles as pregnancy gatekeepers and guardians of fetal health (Rapp 2000). Suzie went on to discuss this further in terms of traditional gender roles:

INTERVIEWER: So you think he sees it more as your role?

SUZIE: Yeah. I don't particularly think of it as my role because that's quite sexist, but I think he sees it as it's not his place, it's not for him to read that sort of thing. It's strange and quite old fashioned, and it is quite sexist in a way. But, I think that's the perspective of it, that's what happens.

(Suzie, 34, Wages clerk)

Women tended to take the major role in seeking out written information and disseminating that information to their male partners. In this respect women can be seen as gatekeepers of pregnancy and screening deciding what and how much to tell their male partners. This perhaps can be seen to have two implications: on the one hand it places women at the centre of pregnancy and screening highlighting the importance of their reproductive autonomy. On the other hand it also reinforces a traditional set of gender roles whereby women take the major responsibility for fetal health while men are distanced from the process (Markens, Browner and Preloran 2003). From the accounts explored so far then we can see that information seeking and gate keeping seemed to reinforce traditional gender roles around pregnancy. As will be articulated within the following section, this was something which was reinforced by midwives who directed information (both oral and written) towards women.

Health professionals and the gendering of information

The UK screening commission emphasises the need for practitioners to recognise the importance of women's reproductive autonomy whilst at the same time where possible encouraging men's involvement (UK National Screening Committee 2007). Despite this emphasis however the majority of male respondents interviewed within the study felt that health professionals 'pushed them out' of their partners' screening experiences, making screening a 'woman only' affair. This included the dissemination of information about pregnancy and screening which took place during routine antenatal clinic. Many men felt information disseminated during antenatal appointments was directed at women only. This can be seen in the account from John whose partner Christine was in the third trimester of pregnancy:

> Well, she (midwife) spoke mostly to my wife, laying out her options and that. Obviously everything went to my wife as well, all the leaflets and stuff even though I was there too. I felt that it was very much about her.
>
> (John, 37, Currently unemployed)

This was reinforced by a number of men such as Rosie's partner Pete: 'No, they (midwives) didn't give me owt did they. Basically, they told my wife all that she needed to know about the tests and that and she passed it on to me' (Pete, 31, Plasterer). Accounts from pregnant women also reinforced this view. Women felt that they were the main recipients of information that was disseminated by the midwife, whether oral or written. This can be seen in the account from Rebecca who was in the second trimester of pregnancy: 'No I don't think they gave anything to my husband. It was left to me to tell him. It's a shame really, maybe if the midwife had told him directly he may have paid more attention!' (Rebecca, 36, Housewife).

In the study women sometimes felt that they were given oral information by midwives about screening at antenatal appointments. However, they often felt that they weren't given enough time to disseminate this information to their partners before decisions needed to be made about which tests to opt for. This impacted on couples' abilities to make decisions about screening jointly. This can be seen in the quote from Liz, in the third trimester of pregnancy:

> When I had my second midwife appointment, she (midwife) was going through all the screening tests. I was a bit sort of overwhelmed because it

> was only eight weeks then and I hadn't given it an awful lot of thought. I had to stop her and say look, I need to talk about this with my partner.
>
> (Liz, 32, University researcher)

This feeling of being pushed out when it came to receiving information from midwives was reinforced in men's accounts on their experiences of their partner's prenatal care more generally. Men discussed the ways in which midwives often made them feel as though they had a limited role in their partners' pregnancy and prenatal care. At times men seemed to suggest that midwives' views reflected a traditionally gendered approach to men and women's roles in pregnancy and screening. This can be seen in the quote from Alan whose partner Jan was in the first trimester of pregnancy, for example:

> It's almost like she felt I was of limited use there (in prenatal clinic), that it wasn't my tackle under the microscope. She sort of made me feel like I should have been doing something more practical like putting up the cot or earning the money to support my wife and baby.
>
> (Alan, 40, Plumber)

The findings outlined here around men's exclusion from information dissemination have been supported in studies on men's roles and antenatal care more generally. Existing studies have highlighted the ways in which fathers are regularly dismissed in consultations and seldom approached directly by the midwife (Olsson and Jansson 2001). However, midwives work in a highly pressurised screening environment where they may have multiple obligations, to women, to their employer, to colleagues and various other agencies (Levy 1999; Markens, Browner and Preloran 2003). Even when it comes to disseminating information directly to women as Williams *et al.* (2002) found 'due to the lack of time within antenatal consultations, practitioners tended to rely on the leaflets women had been sent prior to attending clinic' (2002: 233). It is no surprise therefore that that they have even less time to focus on information dissemination to male partners. However, as this study and others have shown, midwives do often leave men out of screening consultations limiting men's roles in the process. So far in this chapter it would seem that information seeking, consuming and dissemination is a heavily gendered process. Within the last section however, I want to explore one area where this is potentially changing and that is with regard to the Internet. The Internet has increasingly become an important tool in the area of health and pregnancy information. As will be shown in the following sections, this has the potential to contribute a challenge to existing gender roles in pregnancy and screening.

The Internet, health and pregnancy information

Giddens (1991) suggests that we live in an information-rich society in which life plans and strategies have to be negotiated via a complex, competing and sometimes contradictory sources of information. As part of this information-driven society we have seen the increase in the use of the Internet as a health resource (Hardey 1999). This was sparked in the UK by the publication of the Green Paper *Our Healthier Nation* (DoH 1998) which anticipated a government Internet resource, 'Wired for Health' as a source of health information for schools and colleges as well as the public. The Internet has since become a unique medium in which expert knowledge on health is accessible to anyone with a networked computer. As such the Internet has provided a challenge to the doctor/patient hierarchy (Hardey 1999). Better informed patients may increasingly participate in the diagnostic-therapeutic decision-making process, potentially altering the previously asymmetrical balance of power. In using the Internet medical dominance is challenged not only by exposing exotic medical knowledge, but also by the presence of a range of information about approaches to health (Good 1994). The main problem highlighted so far with this increasing role of the Internet in health and health care is the issue of regulation and quality of information given (Hardey 1999).

While the Internet has become increasingly used as part of routine health and health care more generally, some authors have also highlighted the ways in which it has started to be used more specifically in the context of pregnancy. As Lowe *et al.* (2009) have shown, the provision of pregnancy information on the Internet can be seen to complement traditional patterns of pregnancy information. Many printed sources may even have accompanying websites (e.g. emmasdiary.co.uk) and some sites focus on building virtual communities (e.g. Babycentre 2011; Netmums 2011) mirroring the formal and informal pattern of traditional sources (Lowe *et al.* 2009). Women may seek out the Internet as a resource for general pregnancy information and information about fetal development and health (Larsson 2009). Furthermore, Internet support groups may also provide a unique forum and resource for pregnant women (Lowe *et al.* 2009). In their study Lowe *et al.* (2009) found that the Internet was particularly useful for women when a problematic pregnancy was identified through screening and diagnostic testing. When this occurred, women had to look for information sources that went beyond traditional ones. The Internet provided a variety of sources of information for women that could be accessed immediately and referred back to. It also enabled women to be in control of information and deepen their understanding of particular issues for example searching for pictures of things like cleft palate in order to prepare themselves and their families (Lowe *et al.* 2009). Women in their study also used websites as a source of support to gain an understanding of the experiences of others in similar positions. Sometimes women felt that the support they received through Internet forums was better than that given by health professionals. They also felt that health professionals didn't always have sufficient knowledge of particular fetal anomalies (Lowe *et al.* 2009).

Developing on the findings of the research by Lowe *et al.* (2009) the importance of the Internet as a resource for pregnant women undergoing screening will be explored within the context of the findings of this study. However, this section of the chapter has a further aim: to explore gender roles, screening and Internet use. Existing studies have recently highlighted similarities in the amount of Internet use between men and women but differences in the *type* of use. For example, in their large-scale survey of US undergraduates Jackson *et al.* (2001) found that females use email more than males, consistent with a need for greater interpersonal communication. Similarly women's greater use of social networking sites such as Facebook and Twitter have been recently emphasised (Mele 2009). Jackson *et al.* (2001) found that men on the other hand tend to use the web more than women, consistent with their stronger motivation for information. Both men and women therefore appear to use the Internet for the same amount of time but use it differently. As argued earlier, within the context of pregnancy and screening studies have just begun to show that the Internet enables both women and men access to pregnancy-related information (Locock and Alexander 2006). This section will explore this issue further emphasising the importance of the Internet as a search tool for men in particular.

Women, pregnancy and the Internet

In support of the findings of earlier studies women in this context did use the Internet along with other more traditional sources of information such as leaflets and oral dissemination by health professionals. Women tended to see it as just another part of information gathering about pregnancy and childbirth. This can be seen in the account from Joanne who was in the second trimester of pregnancy: 'Well, I did both, looked at the Internet and at the leaflets. You know I just wanted to get as much information as possible, to be as informed as possible' (Joanne, 35, Nurse).

Again as found in the study by Lowe *et al.* (2009), women within this study used the Internet as a tool to clarify or give further information to supplement their existing knowledge about screening. This can be seen in the account from Linda who was in the third trimester of pregnancy.

> Mmm I did go to the Internet because you can find out a bit more there. I was a bit paranoid initially about having some of the tests, about whether they are reliable so I went on the Internet for further information and reassurance.
>
> (Linda, 30, Child-minder)

Not all women used the Internet to find out more about pregnancy and screening. Some women within the study felt that the oral information received from midwives, along with leaflets actually provided them with enough information. These women didn't feel that they needed to search the Internet for more information. This can be seen in the account from Eleanor who was in the third trimester of pregnancy:

> I didn't bother so much with the Internet you know because the midwife talked me through everything. I kind of got bombarded with leaflets about stuff anyway, so didn't feel I needed much more.
>
> (Eleanor, 34, Director of family business)

Again as with other studies on the Internet and pregnancy, women often found informal websites and forums including blogs from other pregnant women more useful then official NHS websites on pregnancy and screening. This can be seen in the account from Zoe:

> I used BabyCenter a lot! I especially like the chat between mums and mums-to-be, but that was more for general information about pregnancy i.e. tips for morning sickness, then for information about tests.
>
> (Zoe, 31, Museums officer)

In terms of general pregnancy-related information, women used the Internet along with other forms of information. However, when it came to information about routine screening, this was mostly sought by women through traditional sources: orally from midwives and through the printed leaflets disseminated by midwives. Furthermore informal pregnancy networks also provided a good source of information for women.

Men and the Internet: a gender challenge?

As argued earlier, in their study on antenatal screening Locock and Alexander (2006) found the Internet was an important resource for men whose partners were undergoing screening and diagnostic testing. In the context of their study men often used the Internet to find out about problematic pregnancies and fetal anomalies. Within this study, when it came to routine screening as showed throughout the chapter men were not overly interested in seeking/or reading information. They tended to rely on the information disseminated to them by their spouse. However, when men did want to find out direct information about screening, they tended to access that information from the Internet. This can be seen in the account from Rob whose partner Chelsea was in the third trimester of pregnancy:

INTERVIEWER: Did you try and find out much about your partners screening, from leaflets or the Internet?

ROB: I didn't really bother with the leaflets no. She read them and then told me all about it. But when she told me she was having all these tests I did have a look, you know on the Internet to find out more about them about what they meant.

INTERVIEWER: Why the Internet?

ROB: Well, I often mess around on it and you know, I just looked at few things that we were worried about you know with the tests and that. It was quite helpful really.

(Rob, 25, Factory worker)

For some men the Internet was an easy way to access information about their partner's pregnancy and about screening. This was particularly the case when men couldn't attend their partner's antenatal appointments. This can be seen in the account below from Ben, whose partner Suzie was in the second trimester of pregnancy:

> I did look on the net but not just about tests but about pregnancy and stuff in general, like what was happening to her and the baby depending on what week she was in. It was helpful, you know, I felt in the dark a bit because I can't always attend her appointments and that.
>
> (Ben, 34, Customer support technician)

An interesting issue arose in one male respondent's interview around his use of the Internet for screening information. Morris whose partner Trish was in the second trimester of pregnancy did use the Internet as a pregnancy information resource. However, he did this in secret when his partner wasn't around:

MORRIS: To be honest, I didn't bother with those leaflets she got. But I did have a look on the net in secret.

INTERVIEWER: In secret, didn't you want your partner to find out.

MORRIS: Well, I felt a bit embarrassed, didn't want to pry too much into it you know but did want to educate myself a bit.

(Morris, 37, Artist)

Morris appeared not to feel able to ask questions or actively seek out information during antenatal clinic but felt that the Internet was a way for him to be informed on the process without having to go through his partner. This reinforces the findings of other studies on pregnancy and screening that highlight the ways in which prenatal clinics are female-dominated domains where men often feel it is not their place to dominate (Rapp 2000).

While the Internet was a tool used by men seeking information on their own, it was also used by couples together. Again men's involvement in this context often reinforced women's role as disseminators of information. This is because men often relied on women to tell them about the most useful websites. This can be seen in the account from Alan whose partner Jan was in the first trimester of pregnancy:

ALAN: Well, I often go on the Internet, you know, after work at night and yeah I did have a look at some of the pregnancy stuff.

INTERVIEWER: and did you look at the info about testing?

ALAN: yes, I did, I looked on one of those NHS websites.

INTERVIEWER: Did it make you feel a bit more informed?

ALAN: Yeah, I think I felt like I knew more about what she was going through. To be honest we did use the Internet but we looked at it together you know at night once we got back from work. She seemed to know about all these baby websites. They seemed to give you loads of info about the testing and also what it might mean to have a child with disabilities. We looked into it on the net and it definitely helped.

(Alan, 40, Plumber)

The Internet therefore is a resource used by men to find out more information about their partners' screening, pregnancy and the types of conditions that could be potentially identified through screening. Some men used it alone and in secret while others used it as a joint resource with their pregnant partners. In this sense the Internet continued perhaps to reinforce women's roles as disseminators of information. However, the Internet also allowed men greater access to pregnancy information and they didn't have to go through partners – in this respect their use of the Internet provides a small but significant challenge to women's roles as guardians of fetal health.

Gender, the Internet and problematic pregnancies

So far within this chapter the focus has been predominantly on information seeking, consuming and disseminating mostly with respect to routine screening. In the study only a small number of couples had positive or high-risk results for conditions such as Down's syndrome of inherited blood disorders. One or two couples in the study receiving 'risky' screening results did discuss their use of the Internet to seek out further information about the implications of problematic screening results. For example, Pinky, an Asian woman who was in the second trimester of pregnancy had tested positive for the thalassaemia trait. Within her interview she discussed using the Internet as a source of information for her and her partner Bihar. The couple explored various SCDs and thalassaemia on the Internet and sought out information on the implications and outcome of such disorders. They did this together. This can be seen in the accounts below:

PINKY: We didn't know very much about the condition (thalassaemia) the midwives and genetic counsellors were great and they gave us lots of information. We did also look on the Internet.

INTERVIEWER: As a couple?

PINKY: Yes we did it together.

(Pinky, 30, Bank clerk)

Another respondent, Linda, also had a high-risk result for spina bifida and ended up having an extra ultrasound scan in order to confirm or refute this condition in the growing fetus. She looked at the Internet with her partner James to find out more about the condition and what the implications would be for them as a couple.

LINDA: The midwife gave us some information but we also looked on the net you know because we were both scared. I am not sure it made us feel that reassured. The more you find out the more you want to know.
INTERVIEWER: Did you do this as a couple?
LINDA: Yes, once we knew there was problem, he got more involved and we searched together.

(Linda, 30, Child-minder)

Within the accounts explored here we can see that men take a more active role in seeking screening information using the Internet. Men were active information seekers in their own right searching information on the Internet. The Internet was also used by men and women together as a couple to search for screening related information. This greater use of the Internet by men (and by couples together) perhaps relates to a number of issues. Firstly, couples use the Internet together because it enables them to search for sensitive information in the comfort of their own home at their own pace. Secondly, men in particular may search the Internet in this context because it enables them to find out about so-called 'women's issues' in the privacy of their own home without presenting a direct challenge to their public image of masculinity. In this context men have the time and space to inform themselves about pregnancy without feeling that they are overly interested in 'feminine issues'. Thirdly, searching the Internet for information on pregnancy confirms the findings of other studies (Locock and Alexander 2006) by reinforcing men's roles as seekers of 'hard fact' and as users of the Internet as a search tool rather than as a means of communication (Jackson *et al.* 2001). Finally, not all men are able to attend their partners' screening appointments and pregnant partners may not always disseminate all information given to them. Therefore the Internet can be a way of enabling men to be more involved in their partners' pregnancy and screening without being physically present.

Conclusion

The focus of this chapter has been on information seeking, disseminating and consuming. In support of earlier studies women in this context discussed the ways in which they sought out and consumed various forms of information about pregnancy and screening (Marteau and Dormandy 2001; Lowe *et al.* 2009). Women tended to seek out a range of formal and informal types of information through a range of sources including oral information from midwives, printed information in the form of leaflets/books, pregnancy support groups and online sources. Women tended to be mixed in their views on the value and quality of such information. They often reinforced the findings of other studies which tend to highlight information disseminated by other pregnant women as one of the preferred sources of information. Nonetheless, information whether formal or informal did play a role in women's understandings of prenatal screening.

When it came to issues of gender the findings were complex and contradictory. When it came to traditional sources of information-printed and oral sources, women took on the main role of seeking out, consuming and disseminating information to their partners. Men tended not to seek information out and relied on their pregnant partners to disseminate information to them. Women tended to read more and actively enjoyed finding out about pregnancy whereas men on the whole were less interested. As argued throughout the chapter, this gendered approach to information seeking, etc. can be seen to reinforce women's roles as gatekeepers of pregnancy and guardians of fetal health. The effects of this are double edged: on the one hand woman's roles as key recipients/ seekers of information, reinforce the importance of women's reproductive autonomy and control over their bodies and babies. On the other hand taking responsibility for information further reinforces women's maternal responsibility whilst men remain distanced from this responsibility.

As articulated throughout the chapter, it appears therefore that a traditional set of gender roles are reproduced in this context. Women continue to be associated with pregnancy and all its many burdens and responsibilities while men's role in the process remains secondary (Markens, Browner and Preloran 2003; Reed 2009). This gendered approach to information and screening was then reinforced by midwives who tended to direct information to women. Men often felt left out during oral consultations about information. They were also not the recipients of formal written information. This tended to result in a negative impact on men's involvement in decision-making on screening. Women's roles are perhaps unsurprising here not only given the materiality of pregnancy but also given the longstanding association of women as mediators of family health. Traditionally within the family women have often taken the role of health facilitator, seeking and mediating health information to loved ones (Miles 1993; Reed 2003). When it comes to the role of the Internet as a source of accessible information, however, this traditionally gendered association is perhaps being challenged.

Technological advances in the prenatal arena have had a twofold effect on women's experience of pregnancy and screening. As Lowe *et al.* (2009) argue the rise of prenatal screening and the proliferation of new technologies has enabled the detection and diagnosis of a greater number of fetal anomalies. Alongside this we have witnessed an increased amount of information about these anomalies on the Internet. Increasing numbers of women are now being made aware of possible fetal anomalies, which they might never have heard of before. Women therefore turn to IT which enables them to consider issues beyond the scope of tradition sources of pregnancy information. Within this study women used the Internet as a general resource for information on screening and further testing. This was used alongside other more traditional sources of information such as printed sources, etc. Women used a variety of Internet types of information from informal pregnancy forums to NHS sites about particular conditions. Women seemed to have more of an interest here on advice from other women posted on Internet forums. They tended to rely more on printed sources and oral information from midwives about specific screening issues. This perhaps confirms a gendered approach to Internet use whereby women use the Internet more as a tool of communication and interaction than specifically a search tool (Jackson *et al.* 2001).

Men also used the Internet both by themselves and with their pregnant partners. They often used it to find out more about pregnancy when they were unable to attend antenatal clinic with their partners. They also used it with female partners, especially when women had received risky screening results that required further testing. In these cases couples searched tests/conditions together to find out more information. Men also liked to use the Internet because they often felt intimidated in the female-dominated antenatal clinic and found it difficult to seek out information in such a context. They felt that searching the Internet at home, by contrast enabled them private access to a previously guarded female domain pregnancy. Three issues can perhaps be concluded here: the first is that men's use of the Internet for pregnancy and screening information does indicate an increase in men's roles in their partners' pregnancy and perhaps poses a challenge to women's roles as exclusive guardians of fetal health. Secondly, their particular use of the web in this context as a search tool is consistent with broader studies on the gendered nature of Internet use (Jackson *et al.* 2001). Thirdly, men's greater use of the Internet can also be related to issues of masculinity. Men felt that they could ask questions on the Internet in private about 'women's issues' without this involvement providing a threat to the ideals of hegemonic masculinity (Connell 2000). The use of the Internet therefore perhaps allows men to be more involved dads whilst accessing discourses on pregnancy that didn't pose a direct threat to their masculinity. This perhaps confirms the findings of other studies on fatherhood which highlight the limits to the discourse of 'new fatherhood' on a practical level (Brandth and Kvande 1998).

Ultimately female respondents continued to take the main role for seeking out consuming and disseminating information about pregnancy and screening. This emphasises the importance of women's reproductive autonomy and choice in the context of prenatal screening. However, it also reinforces the traditional set of gender roles and responsibilities around pregnancy and reproduction. Men's increasing use of the Internet in this context does signal a movement away from traditional gender roles towards men's roles as 'new and involved fathers'. However, it does so without posing any real threat to traditional views of masculinity. The findings here therefore conform the existence of a 'gender paradox' surrounding women and men's roles around information seeking/receiving – on the hand signally a reinforcement of traditional gender roles whilst attempting to move beyond them on the other. In the next chapter, these themes will continue to be explored with a specific focus on issues of choice, time and screening.

2 Gender, choice and time

Introduction

Concepts of choice and time have been fundamental to debates on both the new genetics and human reproduction. For example, some social theorists have placed the new genetics firmly in the domain of individual choice (Rose 2001). More cynical authors however point to the increasing routinisation of technology (Kerr 2004), particularly with regard to prenatal screening (Press and Browner 1997). The concept of time has also been central to debates on reproductive technology (Earle and Letherby 2007). Women's reproductive bodies are constrained by time and as Grosz (1999) argues, women are granted no time or space of their own. As will be articulated within this chapter, time and choice are crucial to an analysis of gender and genetic screening. Drawing on data from the study this chapter will explore the intersections between gender, choice and time in prenatal screening.

The chapter will begin by exploring the issue of choice in women's accounts. As will be shown, women within the study often felt that they have a limited amount of choice about whether to opt for screening, emphasising the routinised nature of much of the screening. However, as will be shown the issue of choice for women is not a straightforward one. It varies between types of tests and between screening and diagnostic testing. Furthermore, ultimately most women wanted as much information as possible about their developing fetus and saw screening as providing this. Therefore despite the fact that most women felt that they had a limited amount of choice, they still felt that screening was a positive opportunity and saw it as just another aspect of their antenatal care. The chapter will move on to explore the importance of time and choice in prenatal screening. It will explore the ways in which women are affected by both physical and socially constructed concepts of time. They are constrained by their own corporeality as screening must take place during certain periods of gestation. The importance of screening timescales, milestones and the issue of 'waiting' – all play an important role in women's overall experience of prenatal screening. As will be argued, time is central to reproductive screening and may act in some cases to constrain women's reproductive choices over which tests to opt for. Finally the chapter will explore issues of choice and time in men's accounts. Issues of choice for most of the men within the study were clustered around men's choice to be involved in their partner's prenatal care, including screening. However, within the study men's ability to participate in their partner's screening was constrained. Men were constrained by social and institutional barriers, for example, workplace norms that discourage them from taking time off to participate in screening (Williams and Umberson 1999). The chapter will conclude by questioning the notion of 'choice' in screening, highlighting the ways in which choices made about screening are mediated and constrained by gender, time and materiality.

The politics of reproductive choice

The notion of choice has been placed at the centre of debates on 'new genetics'. According to Rose (2001), our biological life has entered the domain of decision and choice. Individual susceptibility and individual choice are at the centre of genetic counselling and genetic databases. According to Kerr (2004) appeals to reproductive choice are common throughout the medical and ethical literature on reproductive screening. She argues that the atrophy of the state, the rise of consumerism and individual responsibility for health and well being, and the extension of civil and social rights to disabled people and women are all said to mark a definitive break from the past. The notion of 'choice' now permeates everything (Kerr 2004: 71). The notion of choice and autonomy in decision-making over whether a woman should or should not opt to participate in prenatal screening has been central to debates on reproduction. It has been central to both professional and public discourses (Kerr 2004). For example, if we look at screening policy within the UK, we can see the emphasis on choice. Current NHS Executive policy (2001) focuses on consistency in screening and how choice/consent is offered/presented in all health care settings, with antenatal screening options offered at the first appointment with the midwife, that is, prior to 12 weeks (NICE 2003a). When this discussion takes place, policy states that patients *must* be aware that they do not have to take part in screening, they also need to be aware of the risk of adverse results (Department of Health 2000). Choice can also be found to be central to the accounts of genetics professionals themselves who often refer to the importance of individual choice when asked about prenatal testing (Kerr 2004).

The notion of choice has not only been central to professional debates on screening. Women's rights to make decisions over their reproductive health have been central to feminist debates over the last few decades (Markens, Browner and Preloran 2003). As argued within the introduction, as new reproductive technologies emerged and developed during the late 1970s and 1980s some feminists warned of the patriarchal desire to control reproduction encapsulated in these developments (Corea 1985). In light of this the notion of reproductive choice and autonomy became central to much subsequent feminist work on reproduction (Petchesky 1984). However, while choice remains central to feminist and professional discourses on screening, authors often question the extent to which choice is really a free choice. For example, some authors have questioned the issue of choice in screening policy. While choice remains at the centre of screening guidelines the reality is that whilst this guidance is useful as a benchmark for practice, there are many more 'players' involved in the screening process which affect choice. McLaughlin (2003) points to four categories of factors that influence the screening process: government bodies producing policy; healthcare and insurance companies; medical personnel such as midwives; and the women themselves, alongside their partners, families and friends. All of these issues place constraints on women's ability to make autonomous choices.

Feminist authors have also questioned the extent to women's autonomous right to choose. Earle and Letherby (2007) argue that reproductive control is merely an illusion, in that reproductive experiences often have to be understood within the context of contemporary social and medical discourses which influence the choices and control that women have. Furthermore, although it appears that women are offered the choice to have screening and testing, on receipt of a positive diagnosis treatment of a defective fetus, abortion is often presented as the normal course of action (Rothman 1986). As disabled activists have highlighted, real choice shouldn't be just about women's right to choose to have an abortion – but also to have a baby with a disability (Hubbard 1997; Shakespeare 1999).

Discussions on the issue of reproductive choice have also tended to focus on the routinised nature of screening. Numerous authors have considered how the tests have become increasingly constructed and communicated as routine in order for them to be conveyed effectively (see Press and Browner 1994). McCourt (2006) in particular has raised this in two rhetorical patterns of communication: in 'routine as choice' and 'choice as routine'. Through either type of communication, professionals emphasise that women have choice over which tests to opt for. However, the choice to have tests is often presented as routine, and as a normal aspect of prenatal care (Press and Browner 1997). This has led authors such as Kerr (2004) to argue therefore, that many of today's 'choices' can be said to be encouraged by the state, not made freely but within social and professional contexts.

The emphasis on the constrained nature of women's choices perhaps presents a negative picture of women's control within the prenatal arena. It suggests that pregnant women have no or limited agency in their prenatal care. However, as many studies have shown despite these so-called constraints on women's choices, women do often actively seek out medical intervention in pregnancy whether this is a so-called 'free' choice or not (Earle and Letherby 2007). For example, studies of pregnancy suggest that many women welcome and now expect prenatal testing and diagnosis (Press and Browner 1997). As will be explored within this next section this was certainly the case for respondents within this study. Women were well aware of the limited nature of choice and the routinisation of prenatal screening. However, in most cases they did still actively choose to have tests done – and saw this as a positive choice. Within the first section of this chapter the notion of choice will be explored in women's accounts. As this section will show, women do tend to feel that the tests are routinised. However, they also find the tests a source of comfort in assessing the well being of their fetus.

Women and choice in screening

Throughout the study, women discussed the ways in which they made decisions and choices about which prenatal tests to participate in. Many women felt that the tests were routinised. They felt that there wasn't really much option but to participate in screening. They didn't really see the tests as a choice but as something that was just an expected part of prenatal care. This can be seen in the account from Suzie who was in the second trimester of pregnancy:

> I mean at the first scan they take the blood, do all the blood tests. I didn't feel like I could opt out of that, but I didn't want to at the same time. There wasn't anyone that said you can have these tests, but you don't have to. And I didn't feel like there was that option there, you just go for your scan and follow the room round and you end up in the waiting room to have your blood tests. But like I said, I don't think anybody really would, for the sake of having a bit of blood taken, I don't think anybody would want to opt out. But then I didn't feel like I could.
>
> (Suzie, 34, Housewife)

As Suzie's account shows, some women felt that they really didn't have much choice but to opt into screening. Screening was just viewed in this context as another part of routine prenatal care. This supports the findings from Press and Browners' (1997) study in California, where screening was presented to women as just another 'routine' aspect of prenatal care. However, as the account from Suzie highlights the routinised nature of choice is not necessarily a negative thing as most women want to have the tests in order to know that their baby is well.

Choice became less of an issue the more successful pregnancies that women experienced. Women often identified their first pregnancy as a time when choice was more of an issue. When it came to their second, third or fourth child (or more), women often participated in screening just because they already had with past pregnancies. The whole process therefore became more routinised for women with each successive pregnancy. For example Rosie, who was in the second trimester of her fifth pregnancy demonstrates in her account.

INTERVIEWER: Why have them done?

ROSIE: Cos I've always had 'em done. I've always asked for them, cos when I had him [youngest son], well I thought I'll get 'em done and then they asked me again I thought I might as well have 'em done again really.

(Rosie, 27, Housewife)

Although many women in the study emphasised the routinised nature of screening some did feel that they had a choice that they could opt out of screening if they wanted to. As Emily, in the second trimester of pregnancy states: 'Oh, I think they're a choice, yes. I can't remember whether they said they were a choice, but I knew that that was the case, and I could opt out of them' (Emily, 30, Health professional).

Whether women felt that screening involved an autonomous choice or not, most women tended to see the tests as a positive experience. This is highlighted again in the account from Suzie:

> I think it's just because you think it's routine, just like, you're sort of led to believe that this is what you do. But I mean it can only benefit you, if you've gone in for these (tests) otherwise they wouldn't do them presumably. So I don't know, it was just, that's what you do.
>
> (Suzie, 34, Housewife)

Overall, the findings of this study tended to confirm those from previous research on the routinised nature of prenatal screening and the limitations of individual choice within screening (Press and Browner 1997). Within this study women seemed to think that the screening tests were perhaps a little routinised and perhaps it was assumed that women would opt for screening rather than it being a choice. However, on the whole this was not a negative thing for most women within the study. They were just glad in many cases to be able to have the option of screening for reassurance. When discussing the notion of choice, however, women did see differences between different types of screening.

Women, choice and diagnostic testing

Much of the existing literature on reproductive choice in prenatal screening tends to focus on MSAPF screening or amniocentesis for Down's syndrome (Press and Browner 1997; Rapp 2000). Existing research rarely explores the issue of choice comparatively between different types of screening such as haemoglobinopathy screening for sickle cell anaemia or thalassaemia. One of the aims within this study was to explore both women and men's experiences of both types of screening. In discussions over choice, women tended to make clear distinctions between first trimester screenings and tests for Down's syndrome which took place at around 15 or 16 weeks. Screening at 12 weeks included screening for inherited blood disorders, along with maternal sexual health, blood group, etc. (see introduction for a breakdown of tests). When it came to issues of choice, women felt that they could actually exercise more choice over screening for Down's syndrome than for early screening. Women felt that screening for inherited blood disorders was more routinised, as is demonstrated in the account from Joanne, who was in the second trimester of pregnancy:

> Yes, I suppose maybe the sickle cell and thalassaemia seemed more routine and less about choice, maybe the Down's (syndrome blood screening) has more impact and you have to sort of make your decision based on that. But yeah, looking back, that was when I was more concerned about it
>
> (Joanne, 35, Nurse)

Respondents tended to view blood screening tests for Down's syndrome as more important than haemoglobinopathy screening. This related perhaps to a number of issues: to couples' rudimentary understanding of inheritance. They were able to identify definite genetic patterns in a risk assessment of SCDs and thalassaemia; however, respondents saw chromosomal disorders such as Down's syndrome as occurring much more randomly. Therefore they tended to be much more concerned about those types of tests. It also relates perhaps to the greater public awareness of Down's syndrome in the UK, the issue even becoming a recent storyline in a high-profile British soap opera (Down's syndrome Association 2011). Respondents tended to see Down's syndrome as an untreatable and major disability whereas blood disorders were viewed as chronic illnesses requiring treatment. As will be explored later in Chapter 7 of this book, women also often associated blood disorders with minority ethnic groups so white women often saw themselves unlikely to develop one of these disorders.

Differences in issues of choice in screening became further exacerbated when women entered the realm of prenatal diagnosis. Within the study two women received 'risky' results from the MSAFP screening. One of them Flo, a self-employed Mauritian care worker in the third trimester of pregnancy went on to have an amniocentesis in both her pregnancies. As her account below shows, when routine tests highlight potential problems with the fetus, screening and the suggestion of further diagnostic testing appears to get less routine and more personally tailored to the needs of individual women. Once women received high-risk results, midwives often came to see them at home to discuss the news with them and to outline their options:

> It was the same, exactly the same for both pregnancies, and during my second pregnancy the midwife turned up at my door on a Saturday with a leaflet saying it's come back as high risk (the triple test), and what do you want to do about it?
>
> (Flo, 35, Self-employed)

Flo went on to discuss the gravity of the situation for her.

INTERVIEWER: Was that quite a frightening experience or did you just feel quite matter of fact about it?

FLO: Yeah I did feel frightened because they were big decisions to be had. Should the amniocentesis come back positive, what would we do? And I kind of knew in my head what I wanted to do should it come back positive, so, it was quite scary. It felt like I was quite far into the pregnancy to be making these decisions

(Flo, 35, Self-employed)

Flo discussed her experience with her midwife and with the genetic counsellors which she identified as mostly positive. She felt that whether or not she should have an amniocentesis and potentially an abortion was left as her choice. Although she felt that the midwife had her own personal opinions about what Flo should do in the event of a positive diagnosis, she felt that the genetic counsellors remained neutral.

FLO: They were actually excellent, they were really good. I went over to the hospital and you get taken to a separate department, and we met with one midwife, and she was just, she was really helpful.

INTERVIEWER: Did you see a specialist genetic counsellor?

FLO: Yeah, she certainly came across that she'd had some training. She was very sensitive, really listening. She understood that I wouldn't be swayed in my decision (about whether to keep the baby if it was diagnosed with DS). I felt that my midwife would have tried to encourage me to keep the baby had the amniocentesis been positive. But the genetic counsellors in the hospital were very neutral-didn't push me either way.

(Flo, 35, Self-employed)

In this study, as can be seen in Flo's experiences, women's views about choice and routinisation altered when women entered the realm of prenatal diagnosis. Women feel that they get more individual treatment and support in making choices about diagnostic testing and abortion. This is perhaps because diagnostic testing is only offered to a small number of women and is therefore less routinised than other types of screening. In Flo's case the diagnosis of her amniocentesis was negative. It is important to be clear therefore that this study cannot speak on issues of choice when women enter the realm of selective abortion as there were no such cases in this study. Flo's experiences of amniocentesis, however, do fit in with some of the broader literature on choice and genetic counselling. Existing studies have shown how genetics counsellors in particular are often perceived to be very sensitive to the contradictory rationales for prenatal screening, and are often concerned not to pressurise women into particular courses of action. They do, however, tend to deal only with a minority of cases (Williams *et al.* 2002). Evidence suggests that obstetricians in particular are less reflexive and that individual choice is less of an issue in this context (Green 1995). Having explored the issue of choice and screening within this section of the chapter, the next section will focus on the issue of time. Time was of central importance to the women's accounts on screening; temporal constraints were placed on women's ability to make active choices about which tests to opt for. Time also played a multitude of other roles in women's accounts, from the importance of physiological timing in testing to the socially constructed temporal relationships between women and health professionals.

Screening choice and temporal constraints

Concepts of time have often been central to our understanding of human reproduction. Simmonds (2002) explored medical textbooks on obstetrics and midwifery along with self-help books in pregnancy in order to explore the importance of time in pregnancy. She argues that obstetrics now manages pregnancy and birth by carving procreative time up into increasingly fragmented units which are imbued with the potential for danger. Simmonds argues that during pregnancy women are defined in terms of *number of times* and *point in time* (2002: 561). According to her the notion of time is therefore crucial in reproduction. Earle and Letherby (2007) also place time at the centre of their analyses on women, conception and infertility. Drawing on the work of Adam (1992) they identify the importance of time as both an external and socially constructed commodity as well as an internal and physiological corporeal rhythm. Time can be understood as both 'natural' and 'biological' as well as a defined social practice (Giddens 1981; Simmonds 2002; Earle and Letherby 2007). Women's bodies are constrained by time, and time impacts on women's ability to conceive (Earle and Letherby 2007). Time is also central to prenatal screening. As Simmonds (2002) argues, the medical profession recommends that tests take place at particular intervals in the pregnancy in order to receive the most accurate results. For example, ultrasound, amniocentesis, CVS, MSAFP and nuchal fold scan all must take place at particular times in the first and second trimester of pregnancy in order to receive the most accurate result (see Introduction for details on tests). According to Simmonds (2002) these tests are designed to access the quality of the fetus. They may be seen as diagnostic measures of the *temporal worth* of pregnancy. They help to determine whether pregnancy continues, or should end as wasteful production time (depending on the interpretations of various positive diagnoses) (Simmonds 2002: 563).

Drawing on accounts from female respondents in this study the aim of the following section of the chapter is to explore the importance of time in prenatal blood screening. Within this section a number of questions will be addressed: how does time affect women's experiences of prenatal blood screening? In what ways do physiological or socially constructed notions of time affect women's ability to make free choices about screening? What is the role of professional or institutional time in this context? How do women feel about waiting? These issues will be explored in this section drawing on the notion of both physical time and socially constructed concepts of time. The overall aim of this section is to highlight the ways in which time impacts women's choices in screening, more generally emphasising the importance of time as a central aspect of screening and prenatal care.

Choice and time in tests

Many women within the study felt that they had much more time to make a choice about whether to opt for screening for Down's syndrome than they did for haemoglobinopathy screening. At 12-week screening appointments women tended to feel that they were given little time in which to decide whether or not to opt for these tests. During this process blood was taken and then women were given further information about when to go to their community midwife to have screening tests for Down's syndrome. The discrepancy in time and choice was something highlighted by a number of women. This can be seen in the account from Kerry, a stay at home mum in the second trimester of pregnancy who talked about the ways in which there was no time or opportunity to make a choice over whether to have the first set of tests:

> Well, we had more time to think about the second lot of tests for Down's syndrome and that cos they take place later I think around week 15? But the other tests that happened after the first scan, there was no choice there, it was like a conveyer belt.
>
> (Kerry, 29, Housewife)

These concerns articulated by Kerry were further reinforced by a number of respondents such as Trish who was in the second trimester of pregnancy: 'The first time round we didn't really know what we were being offered tests for. It was different with the blood screening for Down's, there was more info for that and more time to choose' (Trish, 38, Academic).

Time was a central issue again when women chose to have extra tests. This can be seen with the nuchal fold or nuchal translucency (NT) screening. At the time of data collection the Health Trust in which this study took place did not offer NT screening as part of routine prenatal care. However, couples could opt to have this scan privately at some cost in two private hospitals within the area. Two women within the study opted to have this scan. Again this was a scan that had to be conducted at a particular gestation point. The test is conducted between weeks 11 and 13 of pregnancy. Female respondents often didn't find out about this 'extra test' until it was too late to participate. As this was not an NHS offered procedure, midwives did not always inform women about this option. Lucy, a doctor in the second trimester of pregnancy, had the nuchal fold scan. Her partner William, also a doctor, discussed their use of nuchal fold and the various time constraints.

> No time to decide really about nuchal fold. No one tells you about it. It's only because we are both doctors that we even knew about it, knew that there is only a small window of opportunity to have it done.
>
> (William, 35, GP)

Other respondents had found out nothing about the test until it 'was too late to opt for such a test'. That choice therefore was taken away from them. This can be seen in Kerry's account: 'I did hear about that nuchal scan, from a friend, but it was too late by then, I was 15 weeks. I just had to go with the blood tests and hope for the best' (Kerry, 29, Housewife).

Time played an important role in women's choices over the different types of tests. The majority of women felt that they had no time or space to make choices about the first set of tests whereas they had more time to make choices about the second set of screening. This perhaps emphasises the routinised nature of screening that takes place in the highly pressured hospital antenatal clinic in contrast to screening which takes place in the more one-to-one setting of the community. It also perhaps highlights differential public and professional attitudes towards different types of genetic conditions (this will be explored in more detail throughout the book) in routine antenatal care. Time constraints were further placed on women when it came to opting for private tests such as NT screening. This test had to be done at a particular gestation point and women often did not find out about the test until it was too late in the pregnancy for them to have it. In this context therefore the interaction of physiological time and institutional time factored into women's ability to make choices in prenatal screening. It also perhaps resonates with Grosz's (1999) argument about the gendering of time, space and bodies. Time for Grosz is a masculine concept and women have limited time and space of their own (Earle and Letherby 2007).

Timescales and screening milestones

The concept of symbolic time can be used to explore cultural performance of screening within the context of institutional, organisational and professional medical management of human reproduction (Pizzini 1992). Here 'timetable' norms come into existence as reproductive experience becomes subject to temporal negotiations between doctor and patient (Earle and Letherby 2007: 246). This is also interspersed by the physical clock (Adam 1992), the rhythms of pregnancy and the need to do tests at particular points in fetal gestation. Women were told they needed to have particular tests at particular times in their pregnancy. Women often felt pressured to make choices quickly by this sense of pregnancy timetable. In some cases women even questioned the rigorous nature of the timetable as can be seen in the account from Christine, who was in the third trimester of pregnancy:

> Well they do sort of bombard you with information about timescales. This test has to be done at this time and this one at this. I sort of did wonder whether it was really so fixed, whether there was more scope really … but they do panic you. What if I forgot to make an appointment with the midwife at exactly 15 weeks, what then?
>
> (Christine, 34, IT consultant)

There were several weeks between the first and second set of tests. As mentioned earlier, the first set of tests take place in the hospital antenatal clinic, whereas the second set are with the community midwife, normally in the GP's surgery. The time differences between the tests not only gave women more time to think about the tests, it also had more detrimental impacts on some women. For example, Liz, who was in the third trimester of pregnancy felt that she had too much time between first and second appointments, so much so that she actually forgot to go back to see her community midwife for her second set of tests.

INTERVIEWER: And what did you choose to have?

LIZ: We have had everything going I think. Thalassaemia, sickle cell anaemia and there were a few others. But I didn't go back for the Down's or, what's the other one they do, spina bifida! We didn't go back for those ones, but we had all the ones that were offered at the twelve week scan.

INTERVIEWER: So you actually opted out of the second lot of tests?

LIZ: Yeah, well, I couldn't, this sounds really bad but I kind of forgot, and then it was too late to go back. I think if I'd been really concerned or if I'd really wanted to have them done I wouldn't have forgotten about it, but I wasn't hugely bothered about either of those tests. I wasn't bothered about the Down's because it only gives you a risk factor and I thought that would just make me more concerned. If I had it and, if the baby is Down's syndrome then, we'll just deal with it.

(Liz, 32, University researcher)

Along with the importance of screening timescales came the issue of screening as part of pregnancy milestones. As Simmonds (2002) has shown, pregnancy milestones are built into the obstetric literature from the date of a woman's last menstrual period (LMP) when pregnancy is calculated to onset of labour. Medical milestones are built into pregnancy in order to assess the successful development of pregnancy. A good example here is the 12-week milestone. The majority of miscarriages take place prior to 12 weeks (NHS Choices 2011). Thus women often view 12 weeks as a significant pregnancy milestone. For many women within this study screening confirmed the advance of these pregnancy milestones. This was crucial when women either needed or opted to have extra tests. For example, Joanne had had seven previous miscarriages. Her current pregnancy therefore was assessed by the early pregnancy assessment unit at regular intervals through use of fetal ultrasound.

> The scans that we have had with this pregnancy have all been on P2 (ward name) which is the Early Pregnancy Unit and they were fantastic. They are called reassurance scans and it was, the first one was 7 weeks and then at about 10 weeks. I would say probably that the scan that we had with the pregnancy last time which was a 12 week scan was the first time that we knew that we had lost the baby because I had never bled

> and I felt that we were kept in the dark there. But I guess really as a radiographer he didn't quite know what to say to us at that point.
>
> (Joanne, 35, Nurse)

Timing was everything for this woman. The further along she progressed in her current pregnancy the more scans she had, the better she felt and the greater chance that she would carry the baby full term. Other women within the study talked about the tests in terms of pregnancy milestones. This can be seen in the account from Trish: 'With every week, with every test that turned out ok, I felt that the baby became more real and I became less frightened about it' (Trish, 38, Academic). Overall, women were very aware of the importance of timing and screening. While some women felt that there was too much emphasis on the importance of having particular tests done at particular times, other women felt that tests conducted at particular times acted as a pregnancy milestone reaffirming the existence and development of a successful pregnancy.

'Waiting' and professional time

One final issue of time highlighted in the women's accounts was the issue of 'waiting' time. Women waited to have tests, waited to make decisions and waited to receive results. This was often one of the issues that women found difficult to negotiate during the process of screening. Frankenberg (1992) suggests that the medical world can be proscribed as a 'waiting culture' which can be attributed in part to the power asymmetry between doctors and patients. In the medical arena time is a symbolic sign where the significance of the treatment is often reflected in the length of time that patients wait (Earle and Letherby 2007). As Adam (1992) argues waiting is about knowledge and expectancy, and understanding that everyday life is temporally structured. However, waiting is not always inevitable if we consider who waits for whom and for how long: in some waiting situations, differences in power are clearly evident. For example, a patient waiting for a doctor's appointment is expected, but if patients keep doctors waiting then they are expected to apologise (Earle and Letherby 2007: 245).

Women within the study waited to participate in screening. Their accounts here highlighted the discrepancy between public and professional notions of time. When women went for the first set of tests they first had a scan in the ultrasound department. Women were then sent to the antenatal clinic to wait to see a midwife who would conduct the first set of blood tests, etc. This is where most of the waiting took place. Some women complained about the amount of time they had to wait, many didn't even know what they were waiting for. The frustration that women often felt during this time can be seen in the account from Eleanor, who was in the latter stages of pregnancy: 'Oh, we waited so long. I almost gave up and went home. But then my husband said, come on we've come this far. Eventually after about an hour we saw someone' (Eleanor, 34, Director of a family company).

Many women felt that waiting was just part of the process, part of healthcare and the NHS more generally. Most women although they complained, felt happy to do this. This can be seen in Suzie's account below:

> It is a little bit you know, you go into one waiting room (ultrasound) and have whatever (scan) done and then they tell you to go round (to the clinic waiting room), and you just, you see people that you've seen in one waiting room and you know exactly what they've had done because you know that they've just been in for their scan and then come out, and they're waiting as well. It is a little bit of a pain but it works though, because you know, on both times I've not been waiting any longer than sort of an hour at the most. And so it does work.
>
> (Suzie, 34, Housewife)

Many women were aware of the pressures that were faced by the midwives and so acknowledged that they would have to wait to be seen for their tests, as Rebecca who was in the second trimester of pregnancy articulates: 'Yeah, we did wait but what can you do. They (midwives) were right busy. What can they do, they've got loads of women to see. It's not their fault' (Rebecca, 36, Housewife).

In her study Rapp (2000) discusses the waiting period that women faced after amniocentesis. She identifies this liminal period as a time of acute anxiety for women, emphasising the time-framed embodied nature of pregnancy, a period replete with unknown dangers and fears. Within this study women also discussed the anxiety of waiting for screening results. When results were normal women did not hear from the health authority. However, if any issues were raised through screening women were contacted straight away. Women often talked about watching the post and waiting for test results and the stress that that involved. Again women raised the issue of timing and choice. This can be seen in the account from Chelsea who was in the third trimester of pregnancy:

> I hated the wait for the results. You wait to get something through the post and if you do, you know the news isn't good, that something's wrong with the baby. Then you have to make the impossible choice, to have the amniocentesis or not. Fortunately that's not a decision we've had to make.
>
> (Chelsea, 25, Care worker)

Again women emphasised differences between the two sets of tests and the discrepancies in their feelings towards them. Most women weren't so worried about waiting for the first set of test results. They were much more fearful waiting for the results from the blood screening for Down's syndrome. This can be seen below in the quote from Joanne:

> Yes I suppose that the tests that we had a couple of weeks ago which were about the HIV, thalassaemia, you are pretty 100% sure that they are all going to come back clear. Whereas, the implications for these (Down's

> screening), not so much coming to have the blood tests, but I have just found out how long are we going to have to wait and I know that they come to your house if it is high risk. The thought of seeing the midwife at your door, it is just awful. I mean I worry sick about two weeks that we are waiting, and I know I will. But it makes sense, it does make sense (to do it in this way).
>
> (Joanne, 35, Nurse)

Women's accounts then highlight the importance of time; women's choices were influenced and constrained by time – both physiological notions of time, clock time and socially constructed notions of time. Time affected women's ability to choose particular tests and sometimes women simply ran out of biological time to have certain tests. Time not only affected women's choices about whether or not to have particular tests, it also affected their experiences of screening in other ways. For example, waiting was a central aspect in women's accounts. Women waited to participate in screening their accounts here highlighted the discrepancy between public and professional notions of time. Women also waited for results. In this context we see the intersection of time and fear whilst women waited to have the temporal worth of their pregnancy confirmed (Simmonds 2002).

Men, choice and temporal constraints

This section will explore issues of 'choice' and 'time' in men's accounts on screening. As will be shown in this section the issue of choice in interviews with men related to a number of issues including choice over which tests partners would opt for. However, for most of the men it referred predominantly to their 'choice' about whether or not to attend their partner's prenatal screening appointments. Furthermore, discussions on issues of choice and time in this context concentrated on institutional temporal constraints – put simply on men's (in) ability to get time off work in order to 'choose' to participate in their partners' screening. Explorations of choice and time within men's accounts will therefore be interwoven with an examination of institutional and organisational constraints on men's screening choices.

Male choices in the screening context

When it came to the issue of choice, most men chose to be involved in their partners' screening. Out of the 16 men interviewed, seven attended all pre-natal appointments, both community and hospital midwife appointments. This included all blood screening appointments, both haemoglobinopathy screening and screening for Down's syndrome and neural tube defects. Twelve men attended hospital appointments only which included haemoglobinopathy screening and the dating scan, both of which took place at around 12 weeks. It also included attendance at the 20-week anomaly scan. Two male partners did not attend any prenatal appointments. One was posted overseas in the army, and the other was a father of five who didn't feel his attendance was necessary. Without a doubt, most men chose to be involved in their partner's screening. This can be seen in the accounts from John who was Christine's partner:

> Well, I chose to be involved, I mean I wanted to be. I know some dads don't but I did, I wanted to go to as much as possible.
>
> (John, 37, Currently unemployed)

John then compared the ability for men to 'choose' to be involved in their partners' pregnancy and antenatal care now in the twenty-first century, with their inability to choose to be involved in the past:

INTERVIEWER: So men have a choice then?
JOHN: Course they do, it's not like the old days when they weren't allowed to be involved.

(John, 37, Currently unemployed)

The comparative focus on the issue of men's choice to be involved in their partner's pregnancy and screening was something reinforced by a number of respondents. As Liz showed in her account below:

> I think a lot more men can choose to get involved in the process now. It's not seen as a mystery any more. My boss said, in the library that I used to work in, his father wasn't allowed into the old maternity hospital. His mother had to sort of hold him up at the window so that his Dad could stand and glow, you know, seeing his offspring! We've moved on a lot since then …
>
> (Liz, 32, University researcher)

Although most men discussed choice in the context of their 'choice' to be involved, some of the men in the study did talk more specifically about the issue of reproductive choice. Men often wanted to be involved in screening as they wanted to participate in their partners' choices over screening. This is something articulated by Trish's partner Morris: 'I wanted to know what options we had so that we could decide together. Although I respect her choice, at the end of the day it's our baby' (Morris, 37, Artist).

Other men talked more specifically about whether health professionals gave them (as couples) choice over tests. Sean, whose partner Kylie was in the second trimester of pregnancy, highlighted the ways in which he felt that the midwife did in fact give them choices over whether to go for screening or not:

> Yes she talked to us about them. I mean the whole way through the pregnancy everything was left up to us and we could have said 'No' to anything of any importance that was made very clear to us.
>
> (Sean, 30, Self-employed)

Men's involvement in decision-making is something which will be explored in detail in Chapter 4 of this book. However, as we can see from these accounts, the key choice for men was about the choice to participate in their partners' screening and their ability to participate in their partner's screening choices. Although many men wanted to be involved, as will be seen in the next section, there were several constraints on men's ability to make choices about their participation.

The rigours of institutional time

The issue of time has been central to existing debates on contemporary work practices. For example, long working hours and the discrepancies in work-life balances have formed the centre of much of the literature on work in recent years (Bunting 2004). Included in these evaluations are explorations of family friendly work policies enabling men time off in order to be more active fathers. When it comes to issues of prenatal care, however, within the UK there is no legislation as yet that allows men the legal right to take 'time off' work to attend their partner's screening appointments (Fatherhood Institute 2004). The government has produced a 'Good Practice' leaflet for employers encouraging them to enable male workers time off to attend screening (Department of Trade and Industry 2004). However, whether they do or not remains at the discretion of individual employers. Both men and women within this study felt that men's choice to be involved in their partners' prenatal care (including screening) was inhibited by men's inability to get time off work. This can be seen in Rob's account. Rob was a factory worker whose partner Chelsea a care worker was in the third trimester of pregnancy:

> Well, I would like to be able to have the choice to go with her, but work are never happy about it. I have to use my annual leave, so that's what I do. I mean, I want to be involved.
>
> (Rob, 25, Factory worker)

This was related by some male respondents to gendered assumptions about pregnancy and prenatal care by their employers more generally. As Rebecca's partner Bill states:

> Well, it weren't me being tested was it so work don't see that I need the time off to be with her. They think, well she's pregnant not him. Now if I had to go for tests for something medical myself that would be different.
>
> (Bill, 37, Electrician)

As it could be difficult for men to get time off work to attend antenatal appointments, women often felt lucky that their partners could go to their screening appointments with them. This can be seen in the account from Liz, whose partner Brendan came to the majority of her prenatal appointments with her:

> Yeah. I mean, it just seems very accepted that you go to these scans and you have time off work. I think we've been quite lucky with you (male partner) getting time off work initially. Probably in some unlucky jobs it might be more difficult to. Yeah, I guess, I don't know what it would be like if you were a single person to be honest, that might be, if you were on your own. I wouldn't want to do it.
>
> (Liz, 32, University researcher)

Men often wanted to attend their partners' prenatal screening appointments but felt that they often could not get time off work to do so. This lack of workplace support for men's involvement in pregnancy is underpinned by the male model of work which continues to be deeply embedded in most organisational cultures (Lewis 2001). This model supports the idea of men as the 'unencumbered worker' free from caring and domestic duties (Hochschild, 1989, 2001; Crompton 2006), in contrast to the 'woman worker' associated with part-time low status work, the domestic sphere and childcare (Scott 2006; Halrynjo 2009).

In evaluating men's ability to take part in their partners' prenatal care, some couples talked not only about the inflexibility of employers in failing to let men take time off. They also talked of the inflexibility of the NHS around the issue of scheduling appointments. Many women felt pressured to just take the time slots they were given by the hospital, even when their male partners couldn't participate. Women didn't feel able to rearrange screening dates. This again reinforces temporal negotiations and inequalities between patients and professionals (Pizzini 1992). This was something that was felt acutely felt by one couple, Emma and her partner Jo who was in the army and posted in Cyprus. He couldn't attend her scans and early tests because of his work and was disappointed as a result.

> Yeah, he's very erm, even though he's away at the minute, he likes to be involved and he likes to know everything. He had to work, when he was, even actually back in England and he still had to work when I had my scan, which he wasn't very impressed about and asked if I could rearrange a scan. And I said how difficult it is to get a date and stuff like that. I wanted to know if everything was ok, so we had a bit of a disagreement about me having the scan because he couldn't get time off. But he's very involved, maybe too much (laughs)!
>
> (Emma, 22, Nanny)

While some men may use the excuse of not being able to get time off work as a reason not to attend their partners' screening appointments (Markens, Browner and Preloran 2003), many men felt discouraged by workplace norms and cultures from taking time off work for family, or expressing a wish for flexible work (Dex 2003). This affects men's ability to be involved in their partner's prenatal care and in discussions about choices that women are faced with in screening. Time is crucial to this gendered model of work and reproduction; temporal arrangements as argued by many can be viewed as indicators of gendered power divisions in family life (Hochschild 1989).

Time constraints on men's ability to participate in their partners' screening and take time off work was also strongly mediated by respondents' occupational position. Men who were in semi- or unskilled professions often struggled to get time off in order to attend their partners' appointments. They also often didn't want to take time off because of the financial implications of this. This can be seen in the accounts below from Pete:

INTERVIEWER: Would you like to be more involved?

PETE: Oh yeah, yeah, but we got to pay bills! It's hard with my job to get time off, and we really need the money as things are tight anyway. The only option if I want to be involved in her appointments is to take holiday but she would rather I saved this time for after the baby is born … because of this she takes her mum instead (to prenatal appointments).

(Pete, 31, Plasterer)

This supports the findings of Markens, Browner and Prelorans' (2003) study on Mexican men's involvement in amniocentesis in the USA. Many of their respondents were in low-paid employment and it was not always economically feasible for them to attend diagnostic appointments. However, they suggest that the need for men to work often masked the fact that many couples in their study thought men's attendance unnecessary as screening was seen as a 'woman's domain' (see Reed 2011a). In this study, men from managerial or professional classes found it a bit easier to attend their partner's prenatal screening appointments although they still identified some workplace constraints. For example, we can see this in the quote from Zoe, and Dave both 31. Zoë was a museum's collections officer and Dave was a graphic designer.

ZOE: I definitely think that men should have the same rights as women, to take time off work to go to scans and appointments

DAVE: I'm lucky to some degree, I don't have to take holiday days, but it depends on the level of importance. I got time off for both the scans, without having to take any holidays. Where we work is alright, and my paternity pay will be on full pay rather than standard, but then we do unpaid overtime rather than paid overtime so it all evens out really.

Most of the men within the study were subjected to organisational constraints over their choice to be involved in their partners' prenatal care to some extent. This was further mediated, however, by respondents' occupational status, the better the man's profession the more able they were to get time off to attend their partners' appointments (socioeconomic issues will be explored in more detail in Chapter 7). Within this study, gender, occupational status and time combined together to limit men's choice to be involved in their partners' prenatal care.

Conclusion

Issues of choice and time have formed the central focus of this chapter. As has been argued, choice has been a central issue in literature on screening and on reproduction more generally. The importance of women's ability to make autonomous reproductive choices and the various constraints placed on their ability to do so have formed the basis of these debates. The data from this study have further confirmed that of previous research. It has highlighted the ways in which many women find screening a highly routinised process of which they have a limited amount of choice over whether to opt in or out. Despite questioning the issue of choice in screening, however, most women saw their participation in screening as positive. In general they tended to want to find out as much as possible about the developing fetus, to establish that all was well with the pregnancy. The findings explored here do perhaps highlight greater complexities on this issue of choice than previous studies have done. They emphasise the diversity in choice and different types of tests. Within the study women made distinctions in terms of issues of choice – between screening for blood disorders and screening for Down's syndrome. Many women felt that there was less choice in whether to opt for the early testing as that type of screening was presented as totally routinised. Women tended to feel that they were able to make greater choices about screening for Down's syndrome especially when results were high risk. Women felt that more time was put in by health professionals in this context in order that women were able to make their own choices about whether to opt for diagnostic testing.

Some authors have argued that the focus upon individual choice is in itself misplaced, because it masks the professional, economic, political interests around reproductive genetics, and reproduces the myth that reproductive genetics is inevitably positive (Kerr 2004). Kerr (2004) argues that we ought to recognise that the focus on women's choice is misplaced and we need to look elsewhere to understand these technologies and their social implications. We need to ask what shapes the development and application of these technologies and women's use of them. This involves thinking beyond immediate questions about which technologies ought to be developed or not. Along with the issue of choice, time was also important here. As argued earlier, time has been raised as an important issue in other studies on pregnancy and infertility (Simmonds 2002; Earle and Letherby 2007). Within this study, time affected women's experiences of prenatal screening in a number of ways: it affected their ability to make choices over what tests to opt for. Tests were subject to be carried at the appropriate gestational times during pregnancy. Women sometimes missed tests because they forgot or didn't have tests because they had left it too late in the pregnancy for the test to be effective. Women were also issued screening timetables by health professionals. In this sense women were at once constrained by physical and socially constructed notions of time. However, women also saw the temporal aspect of screening as more positive viewing screening times as part of pregnancy milestones which confirmed and reinforced the appropriate development of their pregnancy.

Issues of time and choice did not only affect the women in the study but also male partners. Men had to make the choice of whether or not to attend their partners' screening appointments. As shown here and elsewhere within the book, the majority of men made the choice to participate in their partner's screening. However, this choice was often constrained by men's inability to get time off work. Employers were often inflexible when it came to men asking for time off. This was something strongly mediated by social class with men in professional and managerial classes appearing to have more choice and flexibility than men in semi-skilled or unskilled jobs. Some couples further raised the issue of the inflexibility of the NHS in scheduling appointments. Often respondents felt that they had no say in when appointments were scheduled and that this was done in a way that inhibited male participation. Men therefore often faced institutionally constructed temporal constraints on their ability to be involved. These constraints faced by men in this context as shown within this chapter continue to be underpinned by gendered ideologies of work and reproduction (Reed 2011a). This model supports the idea of men as the 'unencumbered worker' free from caring and domestic duties (Hochschild, 1989, 2001; Crompton 2006), in contrast to the 'woman worker' associated with part-time low-status work, the domestic sphere and childcare (Scott 2006; Halrynjo 2009). As a result of constraints such as these, the gender roles exhibited by both men and women within this study are paradoxical. On the one hand men are becoming more involved in pregnancy, screening and fatherhood (LaRossa 1997). On the other hand men and women continue to be constrained by a gendered ideology based on biological determinism which continues to associate women with reproduction and men with paid work (Lorber 1994). These gendered arrangements while changing are reinforced over time as will continue to be shown throughout this book. This exploration will continue in the next chapter with a focus on the gendered nature of different types of prenatal screening technology.

3 Imaging and imagining genetics

Introduction

Prenatal screening in the UK has tended to include both blood screening and ultrasound scans. The focus of this book is specifically on blood screening. However, as argued in the introduction, both blood and ultrasound technologies are often used together. For example, blood tests and a nuchal fold scan are often used to increase the accuracy of risk calculation for chromosomal anomalies such as Down's syndrome. Furthermore, when respondents participate in blood screening for haemoglobin disorders such as thalassaemia, they also participate in their first ultrasound scan, the 'dating' scan to check the viability and age of the fetus. Subsequently both types of screening are prevalent throughout respondents' accounts. The aim of this chapter therefore is to explore the gender dynamics in relation to these different types of reproductive technology including a more thorough analysis of visual screening and the use of aural technology. In particular, two issues will be highlighted here: firstly, the chapter will explore the ways in which both women and men distinguish between blood screening and ultrasound scans. As will be argued both women and men saw the ultrasound scans as more important because they offered visual evidence of the health of the fetus – the 'truth'. Blood screening on the other hand was often presented by respondents as less important and as relating more specifically to women's health. Women's material contributions towards assessments of fetal health therefore become denigrated in the accounts from respondents. Furthermore, men identified more with ultrasound. They saw ultrasound as an opportunity for them to reconnect both biologically and socially to the fetus. As will be explored, a particular set of gender and genetics roles were then mapped onto these distinctions. Women and their genes were associated with blood screening, men and their genes were associated with ultrasound. This chapter will explore these differences in order to emphasise the importance of 'visual markers' in enabling men to connect with their offspring (Sandelowski 1994), reaffirming also women's secondary role in genetic progress as fetal containers (Ettorre 2000). The chapter will begin by exploring the rise of the visual within prenatal care.

Prenatal screening and the importance of the Visual

As already established, blood screening is commonly used during the first and second trimester of pregnancy in order to establish the risk of women carrying a fetus with chromosomal anomalies or haemoglobin disorders (Getz and Kirkengen 2003; Leshin 2007). Imaging technologies are commonly used for a range of reasons. Ultrasound screening is commonly offered to women at around 12 weeks and again at 20 weeks (Pilnick 2002). Ultrasound is used in the first instance to ascertain viability and gestational age of the fetus. Second trimester ultrasound is used to locate medical problems such as structural abnormalities of the developing central nervous system and heart defects, and kidney and bowel abnormalities (Pilnick 2002). Some of these conditions identified may be genetic in origin while others are not. Ultrasound may also be used to detect soft markers – structural changes which may be transient and have no pathological significance in themselves but are thought to be more commonly found in a fetus with congenital abnormalities (see Bricker *et al.* in Getz and Kirkengen 2003: 2046). The sophistication in visual prenatal screening has been further enhanced recently through the application of MRI (Magnetic Resonance Imaging) in the obstetric realm. This is a visual technology which offers additional information not available by ultrasound. It may therefore be used when there is a suspected abnormality on the 20-week ultrasound scan. For clinicians and midwives fetal imaging has been an important tool in assessing the developing fetus. They also offer pregnant women and their partners reassurance about fetal health.

As argued in the introduction, visual technologies are not only important in assessing fetal health when used in isolation. They are also increasingly used in tandem with blood screening in order to improve the detection of chromosomal anomalies, particularly trisomy 21 (Down's syndrome) (Getz and Kirkengen 2003). As discussed earlier, tests offered in the UK include the combined and integrated tests (NHS Antenatal and Newborn Screening Programme 2010). This includes various combinations of nuchal fold (or nuchal translucency, NT) scans and blood screening at varying points of gestation (see Introduction). Despite advances in this type of screening, visualising technologies such as ultrasound scans are not diagnostic, offering only an informed prediction of risk for chromosomal disorders. Depending on history and a calculation of risk assessment using these particular tests women may also be offered further diagnostic testing such as an amniocentesis (Pilnick 2002). However, in exploring the use of fetal ultrasound we can see its importance in prenatal care, both as an assessment tool in its own right and as a complement to blood screening.

Despite the range of screening tests offered in routine prenatal screening in the UK many have argued that ultrasound in particular has come to occupy a particularly significant position within the prenatal context (Zechmeister 2001). This has been related by many to the powerful position held by the 'visual' in Western culture. According to a number of authors, 'seeing' has become the most important of all our senses (Keller and Grontkowski 1983). As a result there is a significant reliance on the information obtained through seeing. Seeing has come to equate with the truth in contrast to information obtained with other senses (Zechmeister 2001). According to Zechmeister (2001) the significance of ultrasound in obstetrics can be regarded as threefold: it provides information and evidence, it is also linked with fetal management and surveillance and finally it is a tool used to create the myth of the fetus as image (p. 392).

As well as being hugely beneficial for clinicians, ultrasound and imaging techniques more generally are seen to offer significant benefits for pregnant women. As Schuth *et al.* (1994) argue, for some time it has been known that ultrasound tests reduce the stress and anxiety of pregnant women when their results are normal. They increase a woman's confidence in the health of her baby and positively reinforce her emotional attitude. The process of visualisation ascribes the fetus a social identity thus heightening a woman's sense of prenatal bonding. Fears about labour and birth can also be reduced. Ultrasound holds a particularly special place among prenatal screening because many people say that 'seeing' the fetus on the ultrasound monitor is an emotionally rewarding experience (Clement 1998). Whatever their views about prenatal diagnosis, most people welcome ultrasound for purposes of gestational age, seeing the baby and general reassurance (Baille, Smith, Hewison and Mason 2000).

Despite the overall emphasis on the importance of the visual in prenatal screening, some authors have been more circumspect about its benefits. For example, it is important to remember that for many conditions ultrasound is not diagnostic but just indicative of certain abnormalities. Although seeing has become associated with 'the truth', ultrasound offers no more 'truth' than other types of prenatal screening. For example, in the case of screening for soft markers women are placed as being at risk of chromosomal aberrations on the basis of subtle findings in the ultrasonographic image, interpretations that have proved to be misleading (Getz and Kirkengen 2003: 2054). Furthermore a number of feminist authors have questioned the benefits of ultrasound for women; visualisation is viewed as a type of voyeurism which is a particularly masculinist way of looking (Petchesky 1987). The 'truth' that is seen on screen is then placed in comparison to women's feelings which are seen of little importance in contrast (Hubbard 1989).

Drawing on data from the study, this chapter will explore differences in respondents' views towards blood screening and imaging. Initially respondents' views on the differences between ultrasound and blood screening will be explored. Both men and women within the study tended to identify visual screening as offering a clearer assessment of fetal health and development than blood screening, thus highlighting the importance of the visual. The chapter will then move on in the following sections to explore the gendered nature of screening type, focusing firstly on blood screening moving onto ultrasound. The chapter will highlight the associations by respondents of blood screening with women's blood, with women's genes. As will be explored subsequently men appeared to be less interested in blood screening than they were in fetal ultrasound. The discussion of ultrasound in this context will also be extended to include ultrasound transducers (Sonocaid). This is an aural not a visual technology used in the second trimester of pregnancy in order to listen to and assess fetal heartbeat. 'Hearing' and 'seeing' the fetus through ultrasound and Sonocaid were of crucial importance to men. In support of findings from existing studies respondents did tend to see fetal ultrasound as offering them the 'truth'. Men in particular felt that it enabled them to see their biological and social connection as fathers through the fetal image. The argument that will be made therefore is that not only does ultrasound help men become fathers with a more equitable role in the pregnancy; in their eyes it also allows them to visualise their own genetic connection to the fetus.

Bloods versus visual: the hierarchy of screening

Respondents within the study tended to make clear distinctions between the types of screening tests that they experienced. They saw some tests as more important than others. When it comes to blood screening for example, as discussed in Chapter 2, respondents tended to view blood screening tests for Down's syndrome as more important than haemoglobinopathy screening. These types of distinctions in views towards screening were further exacerbated when it came to distinctions between visual screening and blood screening. It was a commonly held view among respondents that blood screening was identified as less of an important part of prenatal care than visual screening. As can be seen in the account from Liz who was in the third trimester of pregnancy below, blood screening was often spoken about more casually than visual screening:

> It's just because it was offered and it was only blood, and I think as well that they (blood tests) are only sort of cut and dry. It was like you have the blood test and they would say yes you've got it, no you haven't, and they were sort of, quite, not minor conditions, but not necessarily major disabilities.
>
> (Liz, 32, University researcher)

The same respondent then contrasted the importance of blood tests with the dating scan. Her account epitomises the contrast of views held by many respondents about the importance of visual screening in contrast to blood screening.

> Yeah, we were just so relieved after the (dating) scan that they (blood tests) just seemed like oh, little tests, whatever. But yeah, I don't know, in my mind they just seemed like they were tests for less serious conditions, less problematic. … And anyway can't you see some the things on the scan that the blood tests are for like spina bifida?
>
> (Liz, 32, University researcher)

Respondents' accounts tended to reinforce the view often highlighted by existing studies on the connections between 'seeing' and the 'truth'. Even though, as argued earlier, ultrasound in many cases offers only an indication of fetal anomalies, it is not in itself a diagnostic test. On the whole respondents were much more concerned about 'seeing' that everything was okay with the baby through the ultrasound image. Respondents' accounts often confirmed the view that if they could see the baby, and it looked healthy, then everything would be ok. This can be seen in the account from Trish, who was in the second trimester of pregnancy:

TRISH: Seeing the baby on screen made it all seem real. It made us both feel better. We could see everything, arms, legs, head, and the heartbeat. We could see that everything was ok.

INTERVIEWER: how could you tell it was ok?

TRISH: well because it looked like a proper baby and once the radiographer had gone round everything she confirmed that it all looked ok.

(Trish, 38, Academic)

As argued earlier, when it came to blood screening respondents tended to feel that they already knew the outcome of most of the tests. For example, because of their knowledge of their own personal history women knew that they wouldn't test positive for STIs. Many women also felt it unlikely that they would carry the trait for either thalassaemia or sickle cell anaemia because there was no occurrence of that gene within their own family history. This can be seen in the account from Eleanor who was in the third trimester of pregnancy:

> Ah yes, we weren't really so worried about the blood tests. I mean, I knew I wasn't HIV positive and I didn't think I'd have any of the other things they listed, you know. Obviously the Down's blood tests we worried about but to be honest, we were more worried about the 20-week scan.
>
> (Eleanor, 34, Director of family company)

As argued earlier, if couples were worried about any of the blood tests, it tended to be the blood test for Down's syndrome. As trisomy 21 is not directly inherited, apart from factoring advancing maternal age, women never knew whether they would be high-risk or not when participating in this test. This uncertainty increased women's fear around this type of screening. However, most women seemed to understand that blood screening for Down's syndrome represented a risk calculation not a definitive diagnosis and they therefore tended to be a little sceptical of their results. When it came to fetal ultrasound, however, women often felt that this offered a definite diagnosis of a condition (even though it is not in itself a diagnostic tool). Fetal ultrasound, and in particular the 20-week scan could be used to detect a range of conditions such as anencephaly (missing brain) which many women had never heard of but which seemed particularly frightening. This again led many women to invest more in fetal ultrasound than in blood tests. As Kerry's quote shows:

> Well, the midwife went through the list of things that the ultrasound could possibly detect and it made me and my husband sick, you know, half a head missing etc. … puts everything into perspective.
>
> (Kerry, 29, Housewife)

On the whole both female and male respondents tended to distinguish between blood and ultrasound screening. Undoubtedly ultrasound screening was viewed by many respondents as more reliable and more able to offer them the 'truth' providing a clearer assessment of the fetus and its development. This reinforces the findings of many other studies which argue that ultrasound is viewed as providing a 'window on the womb' (Overall 1987: 44). Blood screening while important to respondents was not placed as centrally in their assessments of prenatal care as imaging. As will be shown in the following sections, this difference between types of screening identified in the accounts from both men and women can then be mapped onto particular views on genetics and gender roles as blood screening becomes associated with women's DNA.

Blood screening – the gendering of genetics

In existing discourses on reproductive genetics men and women have tended to be assigned different roles and status in the reproductive process and in relation to genetic ties. As Ettorre (2002) argues, on the one hand blood ties are meant to imply genetic ties; paternal connections made by seeds, semen or men. On the other hand maternal ties, based on nurturing and raising children, play a less important role in genetic progress. Thus, paternal, not maternal ties are perceived to be based on genetics (Ettorre 2000). Rothman (1986) makes similar distinctions in her work on amniocentesis. She uses the concept of patriarchy to outline the differences in women and men's roles in reproduction. She argues that while the concept of patriarchy has had a variety of meanings, at its core is the recognition of paternity, the idea that children grow out of men's seeds. Through patriarchy a distinction is marked between 'seed' and 'soil' – between paternity and maternity (Rothman 1986). According to her, men and their 'seed' are viewed as the potential, the 'life giver'; women on the other hand represent the soil, the vessel for men's seed. According to Rothman (1995) this distinction is then upheld in the scientific field of genetics whereby genes and DNA are routinely associated with paternal ties whilst maternal ties continue to be associated with nurture and childrearing.

Given these gendered associations between 'blood', genetics and paternity what was interesting in the respondent's accounts was the ways in which maternal and paternal genetic connections became mapped onto different types of screening. For example blood screening was associated with women and their DNA because it was mostly women who were subjected to screening. Visual technology, however, became associated with male genes because men could be actively involved in 'seeing' the fetal image. One or two men wanted to know how their 'blood' or genes were passed onto their baby and queried why their blood group was not tested along with that of their pregnant partners. Another handful of men saw the importance of their genetic contribution in blood screening through their own direct participation in screening (as was the case for those whose partners tested positive for blood disorders). However, for the majority of men, blood screening did not appear to relate directly to them and their genes. These tests were then seen as less important than ultrasound screening, and because it was women who took part in screening it became associated as more of a woman's issue. In the following two sections the gendered nature of blood screening will be explored focusing firstly on blood screening and maternity, then moving on to explore the role of paternal blood connections.

Women and blood screening – denigrating maternal connections

Some women within the study clearly wondered why men would be interested in their blood screening because after all it was happening to women only, not to men. One respondent in particular emphasised the gendered nature of screening and hierarchy of screening types. This was Suzie who was in the second trimester of her second pregnancy. She queried the extent to which her partner could be interested in her blood tests as they weren't about him. This sums up the association of women's blood with screening and men's greater associations with ultrasound. It also perhaps serves to denigrate the maternal role in genetics.

> I think it is, I think that it's quite hard for men to get involved in the pregnancy, other than scans and things like that. Because I mean, me having blood taken doesn't particularly interest him, you know. It would concern him if any results come back abnormal, but it's, you know, it's, I'm having blood taken out of my arm, how interested is he going to be about that, you know? And I think it is a bit, he's sees it as his manly role to put the cot up, or, you know, things like that. And I sort of get on with the rest of it. Which is not particularly right, but sort of how do you get them more involved?
>
> (Suzie, 34, Housewife)

This type of attitude was reinforced by a number of female respondents within the study. This can be seen again in the account from Kerry. In her account she further reinforces the gendered associations of reproduction itself.

> He doesn't really see it's got much to do with him. I mean, their taking my blood not his, and I'm carrying the baby not him. I mean he came

> with me to those first lots of blood tests but that's more because we had the dating scan as well. He didn't bother with the 15 week tests though. You know, the blood tests are all about me not him, why should he bother?
>
> (Kerry, 29, Housewife)

Most of the women's accounts questioned the extent to which men could be interested in blood screening given that blood was taken mostly directly from women. This is then placed in contrast to other types of technology where men could engage more closely with the fetus, such as ultrasound transducers (Sonocaid) where men could hear the fetal heartbeat or fetal ultrasound where men had a more equitable view of the growing fetus. This can be seen in the account from Katarina, a Czech respondent who was at the very end of the first trimester of pregnancy. She was expecting twins and had only recently had the first set of blood screening:

KATARINA: He doesn't really care so much about the blood tests.
INTERVIEWER: Was he not worried about the results?
KATARINA: Well, he only knew that everything was ok because I told him. He didn't remember that I'd had them.

(Katarina, 28, Self-employed)

Other women talked about the ways in which men often came to the dating scan (12-week scan) with them but opted not to come to the follow-on appointment in the antenatal clinic afterwards to watch women have their blood taken. Again within this context ultrasound as a prenatal check is subtly placed above the blood tests in both women and men's minds. Rebecca who was in the second trimester of pregnancy articulates this in the quote below. She talked about the ways in which men often held a phobia about seeing their female partners having blood taken:

> He came with me to antenatal clinic but not in the room where I had the tests done. He's scared of blood and so probably would have fainted. Anyway, he had seen the (dating) scan so was happy that everything was ok.
>
> (Rebecca, 36, Housewife)

A few of the men were a bit surprised that their partners were tested for STIs during their first round of screening. This tended to make some of the men feel uncomfortable. This is something that Emily who was in the second trimester of pregnancy articulates in the account below:

> Well, he (her partner) was suddenly more interested when he found out that they tested me for AIDs and that, when the midwife said she was testing for that all he said was – 'I bloody hope not!'
>
> (Emily, 30, Health professional)

Overall then, while some men attended their partner's blood screening and did show some interest they did tend to associate it more with women. It wasn't identified by many men as being as important as ultrasound and it was less likely that men would try to get time off work to attend blood screening appointments. Furthermore, blood screening was associated as a women's issue, a maternal role and responsibility. However, the importance of maternal genetics in contributing to fetal health was never really discussed here.

Men and blood testing – the importance of paternal connections?

As argued in the previous section men tended to be less interested in blood screening than they were in visual screening. However, some couples expressed a desire for men to be screened for things like blood group. Some men wanted to know how their genes would be passed onto the fetus through blood connections. Alan, for example, whose partner Jan was in the first trimester of their first pregnancy and who was yet to receive her screening results, wanted to know how his blood was passed onto the fetus:

> The screening is all on her, but I would like to know how my genes are passed on, for example will the baby have my blood group or hers? I mean how does that work? It would be nice if men were offered testing too, to see how they might influence the baby's genetic make-up.
>
> (Alan, 40, Plumber)

Another couple within the study felt that men's blood group should be tested along with women's at the start of pregnancy. One female respondent in particular discussed this within the context of Rh disease (rhesus incompatibility) which often occurs when the mother is Rh negative and the baby Rh positive.[1] This can be seen in the account from Zoe who was in the third trimester of pregnancy and her partner Dave:

ZOE: I think it would be nice if you (Dave) were offered genetic tests for genetic things. I mean nobody, for example, with the rhesus negative issue, nobody tested your blood group or has even asked for your blood type have they?

DAVE: No, my sister's husband was tested though …

ZOE: So I think there definitely could be more genetic tests.

DAVE: Yeah, I think so, yeah. But I avoid going to the doctor whenever possible! (Laughs) But it's never even an option as you're not really consulted about it.

(Zoe, 31, Museums officer and Dave, 31, Graphic designer)

The data from this study support the findings of earlier research which highlight men's interest in paternity, as men wanted to see how their blood or the paternal line is passed on to their offspring (Rothman 1986). However, men's interest in issues such as blood group in this study also indicated a desire for them to re-connect biologically with the fetus during blood screening. Both women and men argued that it was difficult for men to take responsibility for blood screening because it wasn't happening directly to them and it didn't connect them directly to the fetus in the same ways that ultrasound did. By actively asking midwives about the babies' blood type men felt more engaged and involved with the fetus and felt that they were taking more responsibility for the health of the fetus.

In some cases (as will be explored in Chapter 5) men were screened. This happened in the case of screening for inherited blood disorders where pregnant women had tested positive for either the thalassaemia or sickle cell trait. Although this could be frightening (women being in receipt of a positive test result), in these cases men did feel the importance of their genetic connections. This is illustrated in the account from Bihar whose negative test result for thalassaemia meant that their baby would be okay:

> Well, we were upset that she was positive and we were worried but it did help to make me feel important in the whole process. It helped to see that my genes mattered too … that I was part of this baby. Before then it was all about her. Once I'd received the positive result though I felt proud, that my genes meant that the baby was going to be ok.
>
> (Bihar, 31, Shop owner)

Women and men within the study tended to associate blood testing with women because for the majority of couples it was only women who received screening. However, some men did want to know how their blood (genes) would be passed on to the fetus for example through screening for blood type. Some male respondents did participate in screening for inherited blood disorders; in these examples men were more interested in blood screening and saw the ways that their genetic connections were passed on to the fetus. However, as will be argued in the following sections most men were more interested in ultrasound. Men tended to identify this as the best way for them to participate in their partner's pregnancy. Furthermore some men also identified it as a way for them to see their own genes manifested in the fetal image.

Gendering fetal ultrasound – hearing, seeing, believing

Much existing research which focuses on men's role in prenatal screening has focused on their involvement in their partner's ultrasound scans. In particular, as highlighted in the introduction, research has tended to highlight the benefits of ultrasound scans in enhancing men's experience of fatherhood during their partner's pregnancy. In her UK-based study for example, Draper (2002) notes the importance of ultrasound for helping men visualise the baby and realise their transition to fatherhood. In the US, Sandelowski (1994) highlights the ways that ultrasound makes parents' relationship to the fetus more equal – offering men access to a previously exclusive female world. According to her, ultrasound has had the effect of increasing the involvement of expectant fathers in pregnancy and thus has furthered a trend towards family-centred maternity care and a more egalitarian role for fathers. This began in the 1950s, before the routinisation of ultrasound in obstetric practice (Sandelowski 1994). Mitchell and Georgies (1997) in their comparative study on fetal ultrasound in both the US and Greece reinforce this argument. They highlight the ways in which in recent years the sonographer's objective has expanded to include fathers. They argue that this has led to a new clinical niche 'family-centred sonography' which has been promoted as a means of enhancing both maternal and paternal attachment to the fetus (p. 382).

In exploring gender roles in screening, research has tended to highlight a more mixed experience of fetal ultrasound for women. When it comes to the ways that ultrasound enables men to take a more equitable role in pregnancy Mitchell and Georges (1997) have argued that for women it offers the possibility of stimulating or engaging a partner's interest in the baby or testing their commitment to the relationship. However, while fetal ultrasound can enhance men's role in pregnancy it can also have the effect of minimising pregnant women's special relationship with the fetus whilst maximising their responsibility for fetal health and well being (Sandelowski 1994). As stated in the introduction, authors such as Sandelowski (1994) have argued that women occupy a privileged position in relation to the fetus because they carry it. Because women's knowledge of the fetus is embodied they have a tactile awareness and sense of knowing the fetus that male partners cannot have. Biological fatherhood on the other hand is a discontinuous experience; the genetic inseminator role is separated in time and space from the nurture role (Sandelowski 1994: 233–4). Fetal imaging reinforces the biological connection between men and their offspring, while perhaps disconnecting women from their position of privilege.

According to Sandelowski (1994) fetal ultrasound has become a spectator sport for men. It has expanded their physical and emotional involvement in childrearing beyond their biological role in conception and their supportive role during childbirth. It legitimates their absence from work, and helps men 'see' the fetus. Furthermore, ultrasound enables women to help their partners *see it* thereby reinforcing women's roles as gatekeepers to the fetus and the experience of pregnancy, and as altruistic gift-givers (Lorber 1989; Sandelowski 1994: 237). However, it also excludes women and impedes their view of the fetus. Zechmeister (2001) argues that while ultrasound focuses on the fetus, women's bodies become objectified. Visualising the fetus separates and detaches it from the mother. As argued by many authors therefore the benefits for women of enhancing men's access to the fetus through fetal ultrasound is not always straightforward.

Women therefore tend to experience mixed feelings about men's involvement in ultrasound screening. However, when it comes to the evaluation of how women feel about the technology itself, and the role it plays in assessing fetal health and development, women's views are mostly positive. As Zechmeister (2001) argues there are positive outcomes of fetal ultrasound for women, in addition to receiving assurance of the baby's health, the enthusiasm among the majority of women about having an ultrasound examination is explained in their feelings of being closer to the baby. Seeing the fetus can therefore be described as triggering a process of prenatal bonding. Zechmeister (2001) outlines the potentially transformative nature of fetal ultrasound for gender roles. She uses Haraway's (1991) image of the 'cyborg' to demonstrate the disappearing demarcation between human and machine. Fetal ultrasound highlights the fusion of nature and technology potentially blurring the distinction between dualisms. As a result, technology may help to liberate women through deconstructing the male/female opposition, thus resulting in a potential re-conceptualisation of the female body as one which is anti-essentialist (Matisons 1997).

Within the literature therefore, fetal ultrasound it appears, produces a complex set of gendered power relationships which both challenge and reinforce a traditional set of gender roles between men and women. Within this study, fetal ultrasound and also the use of ultrasound transducer (fetal heart rate monitors) were of key importance to men. These types of visual and aural technologies gave men more concrete reasons to take time off work, and enabled them to connect with the fetus as potential fathers. On the whole, women wanted their partners to be more involved in their pregnancy and saw ultrasound and ultrasound transducers as an important way for them to do this. Through the accounts of both men and women ultrasound was emphasised as one of the most important aspects of prenatal screening which provided a window on the fetus. However, in the context of this study, men found that ultrasound offered them a further connection to the fetus. It provided them with the ability to 'see' their own genes, allowing them a window to the genetic/paternal connection. Therefore, within this study ultrasound enabled men to genetically re-connect with the fetus.

Gender and the power of the 'aural' – hearing the heartbeat

Fetal ultrasound was the clearest way that men could be involved in the pregnancy. However, men also found that hearing the baby's heartbeat made them feel closer to the baby. As argued earlier midwives often used a Doppler fetal monitor or Doppler fetal heart rate monitor which is a hand-held ultrasound transducer to detect the heart beat of a fetus. This technology uses the Doppler Effect to provide an audible simulation of the heart beat. This can be used normally from about 16 weeks of pregnancy onwards (sometimes earlier) by community midwives in order to listen to the baby's heartbeat. For respondents in this study this tended to be conducted by a community midwife in routine community appointments held at the doctors surgery. Men were often quite keen to 'hear' the baby's heartbeat and so although often men didn't attend other community midwife appointments (i.e. for blood screening), they often articulated a desire to participate in these routine pre-natal appointments. This is articulated by Zoe and her partner Dave:

INTERVIEWER: Did you attend the antenatal appointments together then?
DAVE: Yes.
ZOE: Yes.
INTERVIEWER: But the midwife checkups are just you on your own?
DAVE: I've been to one.
ZOE: He's been to one, yes, to hear the baby's heartbeat, but I generally go to them on my own.
INTERVIEWER: Why is that?
DAVE: Just because I'm working, I work 15 miles away and so it's difficult to attend. But she (partner) told me about this heartbeat thing and I wanted to hear that at least once.

(Zoe, 31, Museums officer and Dave, 31, Graphic designer)

Women sometimes encouraged their male partners to attend community midwife appointments where there was a possibility of listening to the fetal heart rate. Men often wanted to go along to these appointments because hearing the physical signs of the fetus enabled men to see the baby as real. They appeared to actively enjoy this experience. Again as can be seen in the accounts from Zoe's partner Dave:

INTERVIEWER: And did you enjoy that experience, hearing the heartbeat?
DAVE: Oh, it was great very loud! And it was really fast which worried me a bit until the midwife said that was normal. But yeah it was great actually, really nice experience. Again made me remember, there's something in there!

(Dave, 31, Graphic designer)

Many men tended not to be so interested in attending routine community appointments that either involved blood screening or routine checks such as blood pressure, etc. However, when the possibility of the fetal heart rate was mentioned, this became a different matter. Hearing the baby's heartbeat through a handheld Sonocaid was for men rather like feeling the baby kick for the first time. Women often wanted men to hear the fetal heartbeat and were often disappointed when men couldn't attend. This can be seen in the account below from Joanne who was in the second trimester of pregnancy:

> Yes. He knows why I … Well I have told him why I am coming today (to see the midwife), whether he has actually acknowledged that. But I have said, I have kept him up to date but I didn't really see a need (for him to come today). Although she has just done the heartbeat and that is the first time I have heard that and he would have loved to have heard that so in some senses it is a shame he wasn't here.
>
> (Joanne, 35, Nurse)

Accounts from men and women therefore emphasised the importance of the use of ultrasound transducers in enhancing men's involvement in their partners' pregnancy. This therefore highlights the role of 'aural' technology in contributing a challenge to the persistence of traditional gender roles in pregnancy. Men were more inclined to participate in their partners' community midwife appointments if they were going to be able to share in the experience through hearing the baby's heartbeat. They were less interested in attending community appointments for women's blood screening. This desire for involvement became even more pronounced with fetal ultrasound. Men wanted to go and saw this as of key importance, a reason to get time off work.

Men and the importance of the 'visual'

In support of existing studies on fetal ultrasound many men within this study were particularly interested in ultrasound and wanted to go along with their partners in order to 'see' the baby. This was related by men both to supporting their partners and to their role as potential fathers. The quote from Rebecca's partner Bill was a common phrase used by men about fetal ultrasound: 'Oh yeah, I went to the scans. It's a chance for me to involved isn't it' (Bill, 37, Electrician).

The findings reinforced those of other studies in highlighting the ways in which ultrasound enabled men the potential to have a window on the womb, to 'see' what previously had been hidden from them. For many men it wasn't until the 12-week scan that they actually felt that the pregnancy was real and that there was a live entity within their partner's womb. This is demonstrated by the quote from Paul, Flo's partner:

> Well, seeing it (fetus) there, jumping around like a little bean it made it all real. To be honest until that point (12-week scan) we both wondered if there was something in there (laughs!). But when you see that image, no matter how tiny, you finally realise, this is it, there's a baby in there.
>
> (Paul, 31, Self-employed)

A number of respondents confirmed this view as Kerry states:

> Yeah, I mean my husband didn't really 'feel part of it' until we had the first one (scan), they can't imagine having a baby in there or whatever. But I don't think they (men) can relate to the fact that there's something actually inside you. The scan helps with that I think.
>
> (Kerry, 29, Housewife)

For many respondents fetal ultrasound confirmed that there was a fetus in utero. With regard to the 12-week scan this was a feeling echoed by both men and women because at this early stage women hadn't really developed a 'baby bump' nor had they felt the baby's movement. Women therefore often saw it as confirmation that they were indeed pregnant. Ultrasound also confirmed a baby's health and well being for both men and women. The power of the visual is clearly outlined here as men felt that they could see that the fetus was okay. This can be seen in the account from Joanne's partner Keith:

> It's so good to see the baby on screen. To know its (fetus) ok, two legs, two arms, ten fingers and toes. It makes you feel so much better, I know that you can't see everything but it does make you feel that the baby's ok.
>
> (Keith, 35, Artist)

In support of the findings of earlier studies, both women and men within this study saw ultrasound as a way to validate men's participation in prenatal care (Mitchell and Georgies 1997). Women often felt that blood screening was not deemed important enough to warrant men's absence from work. In contrast, couples tended to feel that the ultrasound was important enough to legitimate men's absence from work (Sandelowski 1994). For many couples this was related to the view that fetal ultrasound was one of the most important ways of assessing fetal development and well being. This is illustrated again by Keith:

> The (20 week) scan is the best way of telling isn't it that everything's ok with the baby. It seems like; when they give the list of what it checks for there's so many things it can check for. It's pretty amazing really and you need to take time off (work) to see that really.
>
> (Keith, 35, Artist)

In contrast to blood screening appointments both women and men saw the scans as an important part of antenatal care that men should attend. While men and women were happy for men to take time off work for scans, they were less interested in men doing the same for blood screening appointments. Again we can see this in the accounts from Zoe:

INTERVIEWER: Would you like your husband to attend community appointments with you?

ZOE: I think I'd probably like it if you (her partner) could come to them, but you've got to go to work. It's not vital certainly, doesn't matter that much to me, but it would be quite nice

(Zoe, 31, Museums officer)

Overall, in support of the findings of previous studies fetal ultrasound was of key importance for men. They wanted to attend their partners' scanning appointments. It made them feel closer to their partners' pregnancy and to the growing fetus. It reinforced their roles as fathers and it was a legitimate way for them to take time off work to participate in their partners' prenatal care. This view was reinforced in the accounts of both men and women. However, within this study the importance of ultrasound for men went deeper. As argued in the last section, men and women tended to associate blood screening with women. Ultrasound, however, became not only a way for men to participate in their partners' care, not only a way to assess the well being of the fetus, it was also a way for men to 'see' the role of their genes.

Visual manifestations of the paternal 'seed'

The majority of women within the study felt that the role of fetal ultrasound was to check and assess the baby's health and development. While men also felt that ultrasound was primarily an assessment of fetal health, they also saw it as a way for them to biologically reconnect with the fetus. As argued earlier by Sandelowski (1994) biological fatherhood is a discontinuous experience; the genetic inseminator role is separated in time and space from the nurture role. However, through fetal ultrasound men were often able to reinforce their genetic connectedness with the fetal image. This can be seen in the account from Alan, whose partner Jan had recently had her first scan:

> Most of time it just feels like it's her baby in her body because; you know it doesn't really affect me. I mean I see her belly starting to grow and obviously she's having all these (blood) tests but you know that's on her. But when you see the scan, the heartbeat, the little body, you know it's real, it becomes part of you, the fruit of your loins.
>
> (Alan, 40, Plumber)

Furthermore, through fetal ultrasound, men often begin to become aware of their relationship to the growing fetus, to their role as dad. Men's identity as both biological and social father was therefore reinforced. As Bihar states: 'When I saw the image of the baby on screen my heart just melted. It finally became real. I could really see what she had been feeling all this time, our baby, my son' (Bihar, 31, Shop owner).

'Seeing' the image of the fetus on screen therefore is often the moment when men become both biological and social fathers. Through this process of 'seeing' men also make further biological connections to the fetus through their own resemblance to the fetus. According to Mitchell and Georgies (1997) during ultrasound parts of the fetal body are often not simply named but are described in terms of fetal behaviour and their baby-like appearance, and their resemblance to family members. In their comparative study on fetal ultrasound in Greece and the US, they argued that pregnant women and their partners often saw ultrasound as a way to see family resemblance. This includes associations with the father of the baby – that is, he's (the fetus) going to be good at sports, just like dad (p. 377). Ultrasound within this study in many ways was identified by men as a means of elaborating not only the social identity of the fetus but magnifying the importance of their paternity through resemblance. Paternal affiliations were reinforced here by both men and women. This was sometimes used by women to further engage their partners in the pregnancy. As Joanne states: 'Oh, when we saw the scan we couldn't believe it, the baby looked just like him!' (Joanne, 35, Nurse).

The biological connection between fetus and father identified through the ultrasound image was something that was reinforced not only by the couple themselves but also by wider family members. In particular paternal family members used the image produced through ultrasound to reinforce the connection of the potential father to the pregnancy. For example, there were cases within the study of paternal grandmothers who identified a genetic connectedness between their own son and the fetus through resemblance in utero. As Emma who was in the second trimester of pregnancy states:

> When I showed the picture to everyone, his mum pipes up straight away. Oh it looks just like its dad! I'm not sure really how she could jump to that conclusion. It just looked like this fuzzy thing with arms and legs.
>
> (Emma, 22, Nanny)

This 'lay' understanding of genetics through the use of the visual reinforces the argument made in sociological studies on the role of heredity in assessing patterns of disease (Hall *et al.* 2007). In evaluating a person's risk of developing disease such as heart disease family history is often central. However, lay people consider the degree of similarity to relatives (in terms of lifestyle or physical resemblance), and are influenced by emotional experiences and closeness to relatives in assessing their own family history. This is exemplified in many of the respondents' accounts here particularly regarding men's roles. Imaging is used to identify paternal genetic connections to the fetus. As will be explored in more detail in Chapter 6, this perhaps reinforces the perception of inheritance being based primarily on physical and emotional ties (Hall *et al.* 2007).

Conclusion

Within this chapter the differences in respondents' views towards both visual and blood screening have been explored. As shown, respondents tended to make distinctions between the different types of screening available. Although the majority of respondents participated in all screening – both bloods and visual – for many respondents, visual screening was viewed as the most important type of screening. In support of earlier studies on fetal ultrasound therefore the importance of 'seeing' and its associations with 'truth' were reinforced. The majority of respondents both men and women felt that blood screening was fairly limited in terms of an assessment of fetal health whereas visual imaging enabled them to see that all was well with the growing fetus. This therefore reinforces a hierarchy of screening technologies where the visual remains most prominent.

Mapped onto these differences in views towards screening were a particular set of gender roles. When it came to blood screening, as this took place mostly on women, it wasn't seen as something that related specifically to men and their genes. It was often viewed as just taking women's blood. The role of maternal genetics therefore appears denigrated in respondents' accounts. A small number of men were interested in the impact of their own genes – that is, they wanted to know the baby's blood group and how it related to their own through screening. Furthermore, there were a handful of men who were required to be tested for inherited blood disorders. These men again made the connections between blood screening and the importance of their own genes. They therefore saw blood screening as important and related to them. For the majority of men, however, women's blood screening was of less interest to them as it didn't enable them to develop a physical connection between themselves and the fetus.

When it came to visual screening, this chapter reinforces much other work on gender and ultrasound. As shown, both women and men saw ultrasound as overall more important than blood screening. Both women and men saw it as enabling men to take a more active role in their partner's pregnancy. It enabled them to make the all important paternal connection to the fetus and identify themselves as social and biological fathers. What was also worthy of note here was the use of ultrasound transducers to hear the fetal heartbeat. While men were most interested in 'seeing' the fetus they also liked to 'hear' it. Being able to listen to the fetal heartbeat was rather like feeling the baby kick for the first time. It also enabled men to participate more equally in their partner's pregnancy and reinforced their role as potential fathers. When it came to ultrasound technology there was a further vital issue within this study relating to the enhancement of men's roles. As the accounts from respondents showed, ultrasound also enabled men to make a more explicit genetic connection with the fetus. Men often talked about seeing the manifestation of their genes in the fetal image. As argued by Mitchell and Georgies (1997) the image helps ascribe the fetus a social identity – and men start to see a 'son' or a 'daughter' rather than a fetus. Furthermore, the importance of paternal genetics is also reinforced through resemblance as highlighted in fetal imaging. Men and sometimes their families felt they saw a likeness between the fetus and themselves through fetal ultrasound. This again serves to deepen the paternal bond, highlighting men's genetic roles as being more than that of inseminator.

As argued elsewhere, as pregnancy takes place in the female body there is an undisputed material connection between women and the fetus (Rapp 2000). This is a taken for granted connection which although material in basis is not directly based on a discourse of genetics. As argued earlier, women are often viewed by society as fetal containers of male genes (Ettorre 2000). When women have blood taken therefore during pregnancy the role of maternal genetics is viewed as less important. When it comes to visual screening, however, there seems to be a much closer association with the manifestation of genes. There is a strong correlation therefore between 'seeing' and biological connections. This is particularly the case when looking at the paternal roles in ultrasound. Genetics therefore has become imaged and 'imagined' in the minds of both men and women through fetal ultrasound. The importance of paternity in this context is not emphasised through blood, seed and semen, but through the masculinist art of looking. This again highlights a complex and contradictory set of gender roles at play in prenatal screening through imaging technology. With men's increased role in ultrasound screening we can see more of an equal role in pregnancy on the one hand, but a return to a much gendered view on genetics on the other. The reconnection of men's roles here therefore in some ways manifests itself as an updated version of the 'seeds' and 'soil' argument put forward by Rothman (1986). However, instead of highlighting the gendered nature of reproduction through the language of seeds and soil, this is now exemplified through different types of screening – from bloods to visual technology. Many of the issues raised here regarding gender roles and screening type will continue to be explored throughout the rest of the book. In the following chapter the focus will be specifically on gender and screening decision-making.

4 Men, masculinity and decision-making

Introduction

As stated earlier, women's rights to make decisions over their reproductive health have been central to feminist debates over the last few decades (Markens, Browner and Preloran 2003). The issue of women's reproductive autonomy was specifically tied with developments in reproductive technology from abortion to IVF (Petchesky 1984; Stanworth 1987). Feminists were concerned that these developments signified an increased patriarchal control over women's bodies. Much of the literature around screening and decision-making has focused on the importance of maintaining women's autonomy, ensuring their ability to make 'informed choices' about screening (Press and Browner 1993, Santalahti *et al.* 1998). With this emphasis, much existing research on prenatal screening has tended to focus on pregnant women as the moral guardians of decision-making. Women make decisions over which tests to opt for, and what to do if prenatal screening and diagnostic results reveal the existence of fetal anomaly (Rothman 1986). Existing research acknowledges that a complex array of factors influence women's decision-making including their partners, friends, social class, race, ethnicity, religion, sexual preferences, experiences with disabling conditions, and so forth (Rothman 1986; Rapp 1994). However, the 'totality' of the maternal role as the source of the gravity with which decisions are made continues to be emphasised (Ivry 2007: 253).

The book has already shown that while the maternal focus has long dominated research on pregnancy and childbirth, in the 1970s, the study of fathers became a popular and expanding area of research (Brandth and Kvande 1998). Several authors have identified a cultural shift towards 'the new father' (Pleck 1987). This shift has entailed higher expectations of father involvement in the care of children. The 'new fathers 'of today are ideally more emotionally caring, develop close relationships with their children and share parental duties with mothers (Wall and Arnold 2007). In the introduction to this book it was stated that with the establishment of the discourse of 'new fatherhood', research into men's experiences of their partners' pregnancies became more common. Men's roles as partners of pregnant women and as potential fathers were examined within this literature (e.g. Draper 2002; Jordan 1990). Along with this increase in interest in men's roles in pregnancy, feminist research began to highlight the double-edged nature of the desire for women's reproductive autonomy particularly over issues of choice and decision-making. Although autonomy over decision-making in reproduction guards women's reproductive rights, it also makes them accountable for any potential negative outcomes, for example selective abortion (Rapp 2000). More recently therefore, particularly in the context of decisions made about prenatal screening and testing, feminist research has emphasised the need to find a balance between increasing male responsibility whilst maintaining women's autonomy (Markens, Browner and Preloran 2003).

Drawing on data from the study, this chapter aims to focus explicitly on men's roles in screening decision-making. The chapter will highlight the importance of men's roles in decision-making, situating these roles in broader debates on 'the new fatherhood' and on masculinity (LaRossa 1997). As the data show, men often take important roles in decision-making, for both screening for chromosomal anomalies and inherited blood disorders. Both men and women within the study wanted men to be involved in prenatal screening decision-making. In fact joint decision-making was the preferred approach by most of the respondents. The chapter therefore aims to explore a set of questions around men's participation in screening. It will ask: does male participation in decision-making emphasise a shift towards more equal gender roles and responsibilities in screening or does it merely signify an extension of male control over women in reproduction? Do women continue to have the ultimate say over screening despite men's involvement? What roles do health professionals take, do they encourage male participation or do they emphasise the gravity of maternal responsibility in decision-making? The chapter will conclude by showing that a paradoxical set of gender roles are produced in screening decision-making.

Women, men and prenatal decision-making

Recent research on women and decision-making in prenatal screening and diagnostic testing has begun to highlight the importance of men's roles. Such research has mostly been concentrated around exploring men's involvement in decision-making for screening and diagnostic testing for chromosomal anomalies such as Down's syndrome. Existing studies have tended to highlight a variety of roles taken by men in decision-making. These range from controlling decision-maker and enforcer to supporter of women's decisions, thus emphasising both positive and negative elements to male participation. For example, within their study on serum screening and amniocentesis Locock and Alexander (2006) identified men's roles as 'deciders and enforcers' as important roles. They closely linked these roles to the themes of men as 'guardians of fact' (see Chapter 1). Locock and Alexander (2006) found that men could be quite controlling over women's decisions. For example, they often encouraged or 'hastened' women into making a decision about testing. In some cases women felt that their male partners rushed them into ending a pregnancy should amniocentesis show a problem with the fetus. Within their study men also took on roles that were less controlling. For example, some couples felt that they shared the decision equally. Other men sought further information about screening, testing and living with conditions such as Down's syndrome in order that they and their partners could make informed decisions together. In these cases women perceived their partners to be supportive.

Santalahti *et al.* (1998) also highlight a range of decision-making roles occupied by men in the screening and testing context. They conducted a study on MSAFP and hCG testing for Down's syndrome on women in Finland and found that men's involvement in decision-making varied. They found that men sometimes made joint decisions with their partners, at other times they played no role at all. On other occasions it was often women who made the ultimate decision. They also found, however, that at times men were very controlling over their female partner's decisions. In some cases for example women participated in screening or diagnostic testing purely because their partner wanted them to. Again this highlights the complex nature of men's involvement in decision-making. It shows that men's roles can be both supportive towards women undergoing screening and also potentially controlling. Existing research on prenatal screening therefore seems to highlight the complex, contradictory and fluid nature of both masculinity and femininity. As Segal (1990) argues masculinity and femininity are constantly being reconstructed in the context of unequal but shifting power relations. According to her, men's dominance and women's subordination is a historically grounded relational system, in which women continually contest men's power. For Segal (1990) the very fact that women continually contest men's power, and that some men oppress other men opens up opportunities for change. In the context of prenatal screening, women appear at times to be controlled by their male partners when men take a directional line on screening decision-making. However, they also (as argued in Chapter 1) actively resist men by gatekeeping information about screening and not acquiescing to male demands over decisions. This again highlights the complex and contradictory nature of gender roles in screening.

In their study on Latino men and amniocentesis, Markens, Browner and Preloran (2003) highlight a paradoxical set of gender roles in diagnostic decision-making. They argue that while men are often involved in decision-making in most cases women are the ultimate decision-makers. This led them to conclude that men's involvement in decision-making was not just an example of traditional male control over women's bodies. They argue that although gender roles in screening may at first glance appear to reinforce stereotypes of male control in decision-making, women ultimately remain in control of the reproductive sphere. This chapter aims to draw on and develop some of the issues raised by this research explored above further. It will explore men's roles in decision-making over both serum screening for Down's syndrome and haemoglobinopathy screening for inherited blood disorders. Where appropriate the chapter will also discuss decision-making over nuchal fold screening, a screening technology only available privately within the context of this study. The chapter will focus on exploring men's roles when screening produces 'normal' screening results. It will also explore decision-making for those few couples in the study when a positive screening result meant decision-making over further screening or diagnostic testing. This chapter aims to move beyond existing studies, however, which have focused on women as the sole recipients of screening by also including cases of decision-making over whether men should also be screened (as in the case of positive female screening for inherited blood disorders).

The chapter will highlight a paradoxical set of gender roles in screening decision-making. It will argue that while men are now more involved in decision-making, in most cases men do not exert male control over women as is often argued. For most couples in the study women continued to have the ultimate say in decision-making. As will be argued, this is something that continues to be reinforced by health professionals in the screening environment. It would appear therefore that women's reproductive autonomy is sustained despite men's participation. Furthermore, while men's responsibility is increased in screening, especially when they are screened themselves, their roles continue to be viewed for the most part as secondary to those of the mother. This questions the extent to which ideal of the 'new father' as equal parent taking on the same rights and responsibilities as mothers actually exists in practice (Wall and Arnold 2007). Overall, the chapter will conclude by showing that a complex and perhaps contradictory set of gender roles are produced in screening decision-making considering the further policy implications of this.

Hail the new fatherhood – men as decision-makers

Screening for inherited blood disorders takes place at a different time to serum screening for chromosomal anomalies. Although practices vary, women are often given information about all screening at their first community midwife appointment at around 8 weeks' gestation. Screening for inherited blood disorders is then conducted at the time of the first dating scan (around 12 weeks' gestation). Men are often present at this screening as they tend to come with women to view the dating scan. Screening for chromosomal anomalies, however, takes place at 15 or 16 weeks and is often conducted by the midwife in a community or home setting. Men are less likely to attend this screening. However, there is less time for couples to discuss participation and make decisions about participation in screening for inherited blood disorders than there is for screening for chromosomal disorders.

Most men within the study were involved in decision-making about their partners' participation in serum screening for Down's syndrome and in screening for inherited blood disorders. Most men felt that it was their baby as well as their partner's and so they should also be involved in decision-making. As Dave states: 'Well I wanted to be involved and make the decisions with her (his partner Zoe) I didn't want her to feel alone. I mean at the end of the day it's our baby isn't it?' (Dave, 31, Graphic designer). The roles that men tended to take were as potential parents and supportive partners. Many men felt that their female partners should not feel alone in the decision-making process but that men should be there to help and support women. This can be seen in a quote from Alan:

> Of course I was involved, it's our baby, I'm the dad and I wanted to support Jan in any way that I could. We made all the decisions about tests together; they were very much joint decisions. I mean she knows her mind and wouldn't do anything she didn't want to but at the end of the day, we're in this together.
>
> (Alan, 40, Plumber)

Men's desire to be involved in their female partner's decision-making was echoed in the comments by women. For example, Emma who was in the second trimester of pregnancy articulated that although her partner was posted overseas with the army, he still wanted to be actively involved in screening decisions:

> Yeah, he's very erm, even though he's away at the minute, he likes to be involved and he likes to know everything, erm, and he likes to help me make decisions.
>
> (Emma, 22, Nanny)

In some cases men articulated particularly strong views about whether or not to have screening. This was mostly felt in relation to serum screening for Down's syndrome. In some cases men's views here were actually stronger than women's. For example, in the case of Dave and Zoe, he was more interested in screening than she was:

DAVE: Well just to check for things like Down's Syndrome wasn't it?
ZOE: Yeah.
DAVE: To work out the risk.
ZOE: I think I wouldn't have bothered to be honest with you, but it was something that you wanted didn't you, so that we could rule it out and then not worry about it.
DAVE: Yeah, yeah.
INTERVIEWER: So did you feel stronger about it?
DAVE: Not necessarily, I just wanted to know as early as possible, one way or the other really.
INTERVIEWER: Yeah, and did you not feel the same?

ZOE: I probably wouldn't have worried so much I don't think, no. But [cannot hear] I didn't feel that strongly about it.

(Zoe, 31, Museums officer and Dave, 31, Graphic designer)

This was related by some women and men to the prospect of termination should a test highlight any fetal anomalies. Again some women and men felt that men held stronger views about this. As Rebecca who was in the second trimester of pregnancy stated:

INTERVIEWER: Do you feel that your beliefs strongly influenced your decisions about the tests, or?

REBECCA: Yes, my partner, yes. I mean with the Down's syndrome, that was a very big test for us, because we don't believe in termination. He probably has stronger views on it than me, so that were a really big decision to come up with.

(Rebecca, 36, Housewife)

Throughout the study there was only one man who didn't seem to want to get directly involved in decision-making. This was Pete whose partner Rosie was pregnant with her fifth child. She stated that his fear of needles put him off any close involvement with her blood screening. This meant that she tended to make her own decisions about them:

> He don't like needles, so he doesn't really want to know anything (about the tests), he'd be like, don't come and tell me owt (anything). I don't want to know, I'm leaving. With me I'm. ... I just make my own decisions about them.
>
> (Rosie, 28, Housewife)

The accounts from the men and women highlighted men's involvement in decision-making. As argued, 15 out of the 16 men were actively involved in decision-making. This ranged from discussions with female partners at home to participation in decision-making in the clinic itself. As Markens, Browner and Preloran (2003) argue men's involvement in the decision-making process indicates that many men want to play an active role in pregnancy and share parenting responsibilities. In their study decision-making about amniocentesis was a way of incorporating men into the pregnancy experience. This male participation in decision-making about prenatal screening is an indication of men's shift towards the ideal of 'the new father' as co-parent (Craig 2006). In most cases men appeared to want to take greater responsibility for their children as both fathers and potential fathers.

'We're in this together'-making joint decisions or asserting male control?

Men were actively involved in decision-making as shown above. However, for most couples it was about making decisions jointly as a couple and as prospective parents. Male respondents' involvement in decision-making was perceived by most women as supportive and indicative of men sharing responsibility for the health of the fetus. In fact, the majority of women did not want to make decisions without discussing the implications with their partners. This can be seen in the quote by Emily, who was in the second trimester of her pregnancy:

INTERVIEWER: Right, and was that your decision or was it?

EMILY: It was actually joint. We did talk about it, we did talk about it on the way to the scan, and discussed it then. So we didn't talk too much about it, I think, because it's our second pregnancy we both sort of knew where we felt where we wanted to go with this.

INTERVIEWER: So what would you say your partner's role in that first stage was, did he, was he actively involved in that decision?

EMILY: Yeah, I needed to talk to him about it before I could be 100% sure what we were going to do, definitely. I wouldn't have felt comfortable going in, I wouldn't have known what my choice would have been if I'd just gone in on my own.

(Emily, 30, Health professional)

Literature on women and reproductive decision-making acknowledges the ways in which women's broader social networks, friends, family and family history all factor into whether or not women decide to opt for screening (Rothman 1986; Rapp 2000). As shown by the findings of this study, however, it is not only women's social circumstances which inform women's decisions over screening but also men's. Joint decisions made by women and men within the study were not made in isolation but were also reflective of both women and men's broader social situation. For example, Suzie and Ben talked about their decision not to have screening for Down's syndrome. This was a decision made which was based on Ben's experience of growing up with a half sibling who had Down's syndrome:

INTERVIEWER: Did you ever discuss with him (partner) about the tests?

SUZIE: No, we decided between us not to have the Down's screening test, but we had the scans and everything, it was just, there was, no we didn't really discuss it because that was what we were just going to do.

INTERVIEWER: So how did you decide about the Down's?

SUZIE: Well his younger half brother has actually got Down's, and we decided that if our baby had, that's fine, we didn't want to know if it has or not, or have any invasive test that has a risk of miscarriage. So we decided between us, and we did sort of have a lengthy discussion about that, that you know, it's fine, we don't need to go for these tests.

(Suzie, 34, Housewife)

As argued at the start of the book the chances of giving birth to a baby with Down's syndrome increases significantly with advancing maternal age, from one chance in a 1000 for women at age 30 to one in 100 at age 40 (Rothman 1986). It is currently estimated that women over age 35 are more likely to give birth to a baby with Down's syndrome than women under 35 (Ettorre 2002). The issue of age was often raised in respondents' accounts. It was another factor that couples felt influenced their joint decisions about screening. For example, Rebecca and Bill were both 'older' parents. Age was then factored into their 'joint' decision-making about whether she should have screening for Down's syndrome.

REBECCA: It was a natural thing. It was something that we were faced with, because we were both older parents, we're higher risk. So it were just a decision that we come up with together.

INTERVIEWER: If you had both felt differently would you have negotiated?

REBECCA: Yeah, oh yeah. He would never say, you know, you've got to, this is what you've got to do and I want you to. We made the decision to have a child and then we carry on and we stick with that.

(Rebecca, 36, Housewife)

There were cases within the study where women wanted men's opinions on the screening and didn't feel confident to make a decision on their own. Women's need for support from their partners was then related to the fact that the baby was a shared responsibility. This can be seen in the quote from Emily:

> Erm, I think what happened, we thought about it more, but I wouldn't have been able to feel confident in my choice unless I talked it through (with him), and felt that he was happy with that as well. Just reaffirm that what I was thinking wasn't crazy and irrational!
>
> (Emily, 30, Health professional)

Markens, Browner and Preloran (2003) call this the need for 'male approval'. They had cases within their study where women sought male approval. These were either instances where men actively got their way over decisions about screening – or where women wanted partners to attend and know what options were available in order to endorse their female partner's decision. In other words, women wanted their husbands involved so that they themselves would not be blamed for an untoward outcome (e.g. miscarriage, child born with an illness). There were no instances within the study where men actively got their way. The latter option outlined by Markens, Browner and Preloran (2003) was more common in instances where women sought male approval within this study.

The concept of trust was often used in couples' negotiations about decision-making. Couples were clear that the baby was a joint responsibility and they should make decisions together. However, at times couples felt that they knew each other well enough for the male partner to trust his female partner's decisions on his behalf. As Liz's partner Brendan states:

> It doesn't matter, it's both of ours. And I would say it would be different, if Liz (his partner) was on her own … but I think we know each other well enough that I would trust you (Liz) to make a decision on my behalf at this stage.
>
> (Brendan, 33, Travel agent)

As Rapp (2000) has argued, men's involvement in screening decisions can be viewed as an articulation of men's control over women. However, this was not the case within this study. Men's involvement in decision-making was perceived by most women as supportive and indicative of men sharing responsibility for the health of the fetus. In fact, the majority of women felt that they did not want to make decisions without discussing the implications with their male partners first. Where women sought male approval it was mostly in order to back up their own opinions. Within the study it appeared that no women changed their decisions due to their partners' views about screening. Again, as found with the study by Markens, Browner and Preloran (2003), rather than seeing male participation as a loss of female control, many men and women interviewed saw men's participation in decision-making as a way for men to expand on their roles and responsibilities as fathers.

Women as the ultimate deciders and enforcers

As shown already, men were very involved in screening decisions and the preferred involvement according to accounts from both women and men was for men and women to make joint decisions. One of the roles that Locock and Alexander (2006) discuss in their study is men's role as enforcers of decision-making, ultimately in some cases ensuring a decision is made. Data from this study on blood screening, however, did not support their findings on this particular issue. Although couples made decisions together over which tests to opt for, the ultimate decision was frequently made by women. This continues to reinforce men's roles in reproduction and childrearing as secondary to women's (Wall and Arnold 2007). Even when women took men's opinions into account, they still tended to make the final decisions themselves. As Kerry states below:

> INTERVIEWER: And would you say he had a say in all the decision making, or mutual?
>
> KERRY: I think I'm the one who really wants to know, if he had said I'm not really bothered what you do, I'd have … I would have made the final decision on my own.
>
> (Kerry, 29, Housewife)

Even when male partners held strong views on screening it was still women who tended to have the final say on whether or not they would participate in screening. Many women simply stated that they would or would not have tests regardless of whether or not their partners approved. Again as shown in the quote from Emma:

> We both did (make the decisions over screening) … He's got another son already and he did (want to know about any fetal anomalies) with his existing son and I always felt that I wanted to know, so we both agreed for definite. Even if he didn't agree I'd still had them (tests) done.
>
> (Emma, 22, Nanny)

This was related by some women to the embodied nature of pregnancy itself. As Delphy (1992) has pointed out, in existing literature the baby is always automatically associated with the woman who carried it. This she argues connects women's identity to motherhood and gives women greater rights over the baby than men. Female respondents' accounts in this sense at times appeared to uphold the discourse of women's reproductive rights over their own bodies. For example as can be seen by Rosie's account below:

> It's my health. I'm carrying the baby … It's (screening) just one of the many things that I have to think about. The baby and my health and if they find anything (wrong with the baby) then I'd rather deal with it.
>
> (Rosie, 28, Housewife)

Men also tended to defer to their female partners' decision. This goes back to Markens, Browner and Preloran's (2003) argument that women often seek men's views in order to endorse or back up their own perspective. As they state, many of the women in their study clearly told their husband their own views on amniocentesis before consultation. This meant that the men were already 'prepped' on the women's opinions. Rothman (1986) in her study on amniocentesis also found that men often wanted the test because female partners wanted it. Therefore while women maintain that they will abide by their husband's decisions about the test, at the same time they actively create a situation in which their male partner is likely to agree with what the woman wants. This was certainly the case within this study for a lot of couples. As highlighted in the quote from Linda who was in the third trimester of pregnancy: 'It was, we discussed it together but I think he sort of said it's your decision really and he kind of totally backed me up' (Linda, 30, Childminder).

While men in the study were involved in decision-making, because the baby was 'both his and hers', ultimately women were the ones who enforced a decision. Santalahti *et al.* (1998) argue that in their study, the final decision often fell on women's shoulders. Despite women asking men for their opinion, women remained the decision enforcers in this context. Markens, Browner and Preloran (2003) argue therefore that women's agency, as measured by having responsibility over prenatal care and decisions is shaped by a mutual understanding that it is an arena in which the woman is most qualified to make decisions. This highlights a shift towards making men more accountable in screening decision-making whilst at the same time maintaining women's reproductive autonomy. It also perhaps highlights a disconnection between the culture and conduct of fatherhood. While men are now perceived to be more involved in parenting, it is still mostly women who take the ultimate responsibility for children (LaRossa 1988). This perhaps questions the extent to which the ideal of the 'new father' is actually realised in practice (Wall and Arnold 2007).

'What if' – decision-making when things go wrong

Several female respondents received positive results for haemoglobinopathy screening and two received high-risk results for screening for Down's syndrome and spina bifida. Subsequent diagnostic testing and male screening for inherited blood disorders revealed 'normal pregnancies' in all cases – as stated earlier. However, many respondents did talk about what they would do if further testing revealed a problem with the fetus. In these cases couples often did not agree on decisions about whether to have further testing or about whether to abort. This can be seen in the quotes from Zoe and Dave:

INTERVIEWER: Did you talk about 'what if'?
ZOE: Yes.
DAVE: To some degree yes, we didn't agree.
ZOE: We didn't agree on it! But we would talk about it, yes.
INTERVIEWER: What did you disagree on?
DAVE: We didn't make any decisions did we? We just knew that, you know, we'd find out the test results first as opposed to falling out about it.

(Zoe, 31, Museums officer and Dave, 31, Graphic designer)

Men tended to worry less about the prospect of a positive result and its implications. Men tended to feel that ultimately everything would be alright with the fetus. As Kerry articulates:

INTERVIEWER: And does your partner feel the same way?
KERRY: No, he's fine. He's very confident.
INTERVIEWER: Really?
KERRY: He says well, you're healthy, I think the baby's going to be healthy as well.

(Kerry, 29, Housewife)

While men often took part in decision-making about women's routine participation in screening, when a test was presented as high risk, women seemed to assume responsibility. This was reflected in the account below from Linda:

> The first pregnancy I had a high result come back on the spina bifida one and it was just awful … I was due to see the midwife the next week or something, but it was just really, you know, it made both of us really worry and stuff. But I felt particularly anxious, you know because it's my body. But then, I had the scan and everything was fine.
>
> (Linda, 30, Childminder)

In these cases women were often concerned not only that the baby might be diagnosed with a fetal anomaly; they were also concerned that any diagnostic testing may lead to miscarriage. As argued previously, both CVS and amniocentesis are invasive procedures which carry the risk of miscarriage (Pilnick 2002). Linda for example who received a 'risky' screening result for spina bifida and was asked to participate in further ultrasound screening, was worried about the risk of miscarriage.

LINDA: Because I've had miscarriages in the past, I was just anxious, too anxious to do anything. And I didn't have all of the blood tests this time.

INTERVIEWER: Have you had them in the past?

LINDA: Yeah, I did for the first one, first one I had kind of everything, and I wanted all the tests. And me and my partner agreed on it. Erm, then we had a load of miscarriages and then after that well I thought I don't want the tests because then I'd have to, you know, possibly decide to get rid of the baby and the same with this one, I didn't want all the tests.

(Linda, 30, Childminder)

Again though, women tended to make the final decisions about screening and further diagnostic testing for chromosomal anomalies. Women felt that ultimately this was their domain and men would not dare interfere with them. This was reflected in the quote by Emma:

> Yeah. My partner didn't say, and I don't think he will say that oh yeah, if it were I'd want you to get rid of it. Because I think that he knows I'm strong willed and no matter what he said I wouldn't listen. So I think he just, to not cause arguments he just didn't say. So obviously if it did come back, obviously we hope it doesn't, but if they do come back and they're positive then I don't know what his reactions going to be. Because I'm not sure whether he just wouldn't dare say 'this is what I want you to do'. So, obviously, time will tell.
>
> (Emma, 22, Nanny)

In the case of further screening for inherited blood disorders decisions tended to be jointly made between women and men. When women tested positive for either sickle cell or thalassaemia, the simplest way to confirm or refute a diagnosis was to test male partners for the genetic trait. If men tested negative for the trait then the fetus would not develop either condition. Therefore it was crucial to enlist men in further screening. Should men not agree to participate then a woman would be asked to participate in diagnostic testing which as discussed earlier carries a risk of miscarriage. Within this study two men were involved in screening for thalassaemia, and one man was involved in screening for sickle cell anaemia. Both women and men were involved in decision-making over male participation. In most cases men took it for granted that they would be screened. This can be seen in the quote from Bihar whose wife Pinky was in the second trimester of pregnancy:

> Well, I went with her for the screening. When we got the results, like, that she was positive, it was a no brainer of course I were gonna be tested. We didn't really talk about it, just did it.
>
> (Bihar, 31, Shop owner)

When it came to screening or diagnostic testing for chromosomal anomalies such as Down's syndrome the focus was on women's bodies. Men therefore tended to defer to their female partners' decisions. With regards to screening for inherited blood disorders, where there was a positive result, men's bodies were also subjected to screening. This changed the gender dynamics from a focus on the discourse of women's reproductive rights over their own body, to joint responsibilities of parents. The notion of joint decision-making therefore became central. As Jameela's partner Tunde articulates: 'Well, it involved both of us so it was both our decision. If it was just happening to her then things may have been different' (Tunde, 37, Psychiatrist).

The majority of male partners were happy to be screened and all received normal screening results. Paul, whose partner Flo received a border-line test for thalassaemia, was the only male respondent not to be screened. This couple decided jointly that he would not be tested. This was because her test was only border-line, and he was ethnically white, and so they felt there was little chance of him being a carrier. As Paul's quote shows:

INTERVIEWER: So, how did you reach the decision not to be screened?

PAUL: Well we talked about it and made the decision together as a couple but as I said earlier, we didn't think there was too much chance of me having it (thalassaemia) as I'm white so we decided against it.

(Paul, 31, Self-employed)

Again, as with decisions made over routine screening men were happy to be involved and make decisions with their partner. However, they also respected that their female partner had the ultimate say over whether or not men should be tested.

Two sets of couples in the study opted to have a nuchal fold scan. As argued previously, this type of screening was not available on the NHS in the health trust where this study was conducted. Couples therefore had to opt to pay and have the scan privately if they wanted to participate in this type of screening. There were no specific personal medical reasons as to why these couples opted for the test. For both couples, age factored into the decision-making process. Both women who opted for the scan were aged over 30 and felt their chances of carrying a baby with a chromosomal anomaly were higher. They wanted to obtain greater reassurance than the triple blood test could provide them with. However, at the same time they did not want to opt for more invasive diagnostic procedures such as CVS or amniocentesis. The decision-making process for these two couples differed. For one of the couples William and Lucy, William had actually been the one to encourage Lucy to have the scan. William was a GP and had spent a lot of time researching different screening tests (see Chapter 1). In the case of the other couple Eleanor and Ed, it was Eleanor in particular who wanted the scan. She had found out about it from friends and initiated the decision to participate in it. As she states below: 'Well, it was me really that wanted it done. I mean he went along with my wishes really. To be honest, he didn't know anything about it till I told him' (Eleanor, 34, Director of family company).

Around half of the respondents in the study by Santalahti *et al.* (1998) mentioned partners in decision-making for diagnostic testing. Again male roles varied, from mutual decision-making, to male withdrawal, to men being supportive stating their opinion but leaving it up to women to make the ultimate decision. Subsequent decisions made about abortion were mostly made jointly. Within this study when it comes to diagnostic testing for chromosomal anomalies and the threat of 'what if' women again seem to take a greater role in decision-making. While roles in decision-making were somewhat varied when it came to the option of whether to have the extra nuchal fold test, or where there was the possibility of women being subjected to invasive further diagnostic testing, then women tended to assume the lead role in decision-making. Here men and women appear to distinguish between the goals and responsibilities of shared parenting and women's rights over their own bodies (Markens, Browner and Preloran 2003). This is because amniocentesis takes place on women's bodies and carries with it a set of potential risks, for example miscarriage. Where further decisions were needed for screening for inherited blood disorders (which would require male participation), then the decision continued to be more of a joint one. In these cases women's bodies were no longer directly the focus of screening and testing, but bother partners had to be tested. With this type of screening the emphasis on decision-making as parents and as a couple was paramount.

Health policy and practice: a reinforcement of maternal responsibility?

As can be seen in the accounts above men did take a significant role in decision-making over screening. Women and men both wanted men to take an active role as supportive partners, as potential fathers and as possible participants in the case of positive screening for inherited blood disorders. However, as also shown by the accounts above, while women wanted men's involvement in decision-making, overall it was women who tended to decide and enforce decisions on most screening with the exception of cases where men were also screened. Men's roles as fathers are then placed as secondary to the gravity of the maternal role (Wall and Arnold 2007). Within this last section of this chapter, I want to explore the ways in which health professionals and health policy either support or refute men's participation in decision-making.

The UK screening commission gives clear guidelines to midwives and screening professionals when it comes to male participation in screening decision-making. It emphasises the need for practitioners to recognise the importance of women's reproductive autonomy whilst at the same time where possible encouraging men's involvement (UK National Screening Committee 2007).

> The decision whether to undergo screening belongs to the woman: however the National Programme Centre supports and encourages her to seek the views of her husband/partner.
>
> (UK National Screening Committee 2007: 44)

Despite this emphasis in policy on encouraging women to talk to their partners about decision-making, the majority of male respondents interviewed within the study felt that health professionals 'pushed them out' of their partners' screening decisions, making screening a 'woman only' affair. As stated by Bill, whose partner Rebecca was in the second trimester of pregnancy: 'I wanted to be involved but she (midwife) made it blatantly obvious that she wanted me out of the room' (Bill, 37, Electrician).

Men's exclusion from the screening experience was felt most keenly around decision-making, and this was found to be upsetting for pregnant women and their male partners. As shown within this chapter, most female respondents wanted to make decisions with their partners as a couple but sometimes found that midwives saw men as having a limited role in the process. One of the female respondents Liz (as articulated in Chapter 2) felt that at an early antenatal appointment the midwife pushed her into making decisions about screening without giving her the chance to talk to her partner about them. The quote from Liz highlights this again:

> And she (midwife) was ticking these boxes (for tests), and I was like oh no, I'm not going to make that decision right now I want to talk to my partner … But it's almost as if she (midwife) felt his views were of little importance.
>
> (Liz, 32, University researcher)

This highlights the significance of temporal constraints on couples screening decision-making as already discussed in Chapter 2. Women have a limited amount of time to make decisions about screening; furthermore, midwives themselves are also subject to time constraints in the highly pressurised screening environment. Therefore women often do not have time to make decisions with their partners. Men also discussed the ways in which midwives often made them feel as though they had a limited role in their partners' decision-making. Flo's partner Paul articulates this in the quote below:

> On the whole the midwives were great especially with the amniocentesis, but I did feel that early on when we were deciding about tests we'd go for the focus was on her not me. The midwife did make it clear that this wasn't about me and my views. I did feel pretty sidelined at that point to be honest.
>
> (Paul, 31, Self-employed)

As discussed in Chapter 1, this exclusion of fathers from decision-making reflects how they are regularly dismissed in consultations and seldom approached directly by the midwife (Olsson and Jansson 2001). Midwives are of course in a difficult position as they must encourage male participation whilst also ensuring women's reproductive choice and autonomy, all within the context of a highly pressurised screening environment where they may have multiple obligations, to women, to their employer, to colleagues and various other agencies (Levy 1999; Markens, Browner and Preloran 2003). It is no surprise therefore that that they have little time to focus on their interactions with male partners. However, as this study and others have shown, midwives do often leave men out of screening consultations suggesting almost that men's roles in the reproductive process are of limited consequence. This then appears to enforce the gravity of maternal responsibility over decision-making, and reinforces women's roles as the ultimate decision-maker and enforcer.

Conclusion – gender parity in decision-making

Men's involvement in decision-making in screening is significant for both men and women. Respondents in the study expressed a strong desire to make decisions jointly as potential parents. Men also want to be involved to share responsibility and support their partners. This undoubtedly lends weight to the ideal of the 'new father' who shares parenting responsibility with mothers both prenatally and beyond. In fact, as the accounts from respondents here show, fostering men's involvement in decision-making over screening is a way of enabling men to be more involved as partners and potential fathers. It is also a way of making men more accountable for the health of the fetus. As the accounts show, there is some variation in men's involvement in the different types of screening. Men tended to be involved with decision-making for routine screening for both serum screening for chromosomal anomalies and for blood screening for inherited blood disorders. However, when things went wrong women assumed ultimate responsibility in the case of screening for chromosomal anomalies. However, in the case of inherited blood disorders, when women received a positive result and men were asked to be screened, decisions remained joint ones. This perhaps can be related to the embodied nature of screening, and the distinctions that respondents make over women's reproductive rights over their own bodies and couples' joint rights as potential parents (Markens, Browner and Preloran 2003).

When it comes to male partners' involvement some authors have argued that this can be viewed as an extension of male control over women in the reproductive sphere (Rapp 2000). However, this didn't seem to be the case in this study. The majority of female respondents welcomed male participation. Where women sought 'male approval' for their own decisions on screening, this was not so that men could alter or reinforce a decision, but rather so that men could approve women's existing decisions (Markens, Browner and

Preloran 2003). This produces a paradoxical set of gender roles. On the one hand women's accounts of wanting and needing 'male approval' seem to validate the stereotypical patriarchal model of decision-making. On the other hand, despite the fact that women said they would not pursue a course of prenatal action without their partners' say so, they did not appear to passively acquiesce to their partners' expectations either. Women in fact were the ones who ultimately made the decisions (Markens, Browner and Preloran 2003). Decision-making therefore can be seen to involve a complex process of gendered negotiations which included both manipulation and resistance by both women and men (Rapp 2000).

In evaluating men's roles in screening decision-making then can we see them as equal to women's? Men's roles here certainly indicate a shift towards the ideal of the 'new father' and more equalitarian roles in parenting. Men do want to be more involved in reproductive decision-making, both as supportive partners and as potential fathers. However, their involvement does not signal truly equal roles between men and women. Whilst men's roles in decision-making are seen as important they are still secondary to women's roles as mothers. This is something that is supported by wider culture and is reflected in biomedical discourse itself. Wall and Arnold (2007) for example highlight the ways in which the idea of 'the new fatherhood' is in fact an ideal which is yet to be fully realised and practised by most fathers. While cultural understandings of both fatherhood and masculinity are multiple, fluid and changing (Lupton and Barclay 1997), the idea of fathers who are as equally involved with childrearing as mothers continues to clash with the hegemonic cultural ideals of masculinity (Connell 2000). As discussed in Chapter 2 men's roles as breadwinners are still of central importance to cultural understandings over fatherhood. Whilst there is a shift towards the idea of the caring dad, this continues to be interwoven with the dominant idea of man as the breadwinner (Wall and Arnold 2007). This discrepancy between the culture and practice of fatherhood certainly does help to understand men's roles in screening within this study.

Men's secondary role as fathers in screening decision-making is further reinforced by medical professionals in the screening setting. As accounts from both men and women showed, health professionals reinforced women's roles as decision-makers and actually pushed men out of the decision-making process. There are of course reasons why midwives focus on women's decisions. Their duty of care is to pregnant women and maintaining reproductive autonomy and choice for these women. There are cases for example where men's participation in the screening consultation is not beneficial to pregnant women, as shown in studies on prenatal care and domestic violence (e.g. Stenson *et al.* 2005). Midwives therefore must make decisions about men's participation on a case by case basis upholding the notion of women's reproductive 'choice' (Markens, Browner and Preloran 2003). However, while midwives may be protecting women's reproductive autonomy in this context, they are also systematically reinforcing traditional gender roles. According to

Vosler and Burst (1993) midwives are a profession predominantly composed of women, serving the health needs of women in a health care system that has been historically dominated by men. Midwives try to work in the interests of the women they serve whilst also being constrained by a medical system which continues to reinforce a traditional gender division of labour in the reproductive sphere. This traditional gender ideology does not encourage midwives to acknowledge the increasing importance of men's roles as fathers, thus questioning the extent to which the ideal of the 'new father' as argued in Chapter 2, has been acknowledged by wider institutions and organisations (Wall and Arnold 2007).

It is of course imperative that women do still have reproductive autonomy in screening decision-making. Women are the ones who carry children and take the major roles in rearing children so the focus of reproductive decision-making should be on them. However, as accounts from this and other studies show, this does not need to come at a cost of relegating men. Both women and men on the whole want men to be more involved in screening decision-making. Where appropriate therefore, and where time allows it, women should be encouraged by health professionals to seek the views of their partners. Data from this study show that the UK guidelines for men's involvement in decision-making are appropriate for supporting men's roles in screening if followed correctly by screening practitioners. They appear to ensure the twin feminist goals of maintaining women's reproductive autonomy whilst also encouraging women to involve their partners – where possible to enable joint responsibility and accountability for the health of the fetus. Within the next section the issue of gender and responsibility and accountability will be explored in more detail through a focus on the production of so-called 'good and bad genes'.

5 Gendering 'good' and 'bad' genes

Introduction

Distinctions between so-called 'good' and 'bad' genes or 'normal' and 'defective genes', have most commonly been associated with the eugenics movement prevalent during the first half of the twentieth century. This movement which prospered in both the UK and US focused on the improvement of the human race through better breeding. In order to achieve a supposedly 'genetically fitter' human race, eugenic hygiene policies were implemented across Europe and the US. These included identifying 'genetic defectives' and controlling their procreation and assimilation into society through marriage and immigration laws as well as sterilisation of undesirables (Conrad and Gabe 1999). As pointed out by several authors the application of such policies had a clear a racial and class bias in identifying socially undesirable traits. For example, the feeble minded and those with limited moral sense or repeated criminal behaviour were targeted (Conrad and Gabe 1999;, Pilnick 2002). The poor and those identified as immigrants were encouraged not to reproduce. The genetically fit on the other hand with desirable social traits were encouraged to reproduce. Despite the fact that the eugenics movement was in decline by the 1940s, many have raised concerns that the spectre of eugenics continues to cast a shadow over the new genetics (Conrad and Gabe 1999; Pilnick 2002).

Since the emergence of the Human Genome project in the 1980s we have witnessed great advances in the new genetics. The aim of the Genome Project was to find the chemical genetic base for the 4000 or so genetic diseases that affect humans, as well as to identify genetic links with diseases in the hope of creating new preventions and cures (Conrad 1997). Through the emergence and development of the genome project we have been able to make great advances in science and medicine through the identification and subsequent screening of a number of genes from the BRCA1 gene, to Huntingdon's disease and cystic fibrosis. However, while there may be benefits to such developments in genetics sociologists have raised a number of concerns. As Conrad and Gabe (1999) argue while the new genetics is more medical, involves individual choice and has not led to overtly state policies, the pall of eugenic history is reflected in anxieties about genetics. Duster (1990) for example has raised concerns over the discriminatory nature of the selective screening practices for inherited genetic disorders specifically distributed by race and ethnicity. Duster (1990) does not suggest that we are back to the open and malevolent forms of eugenics, but rather suggests that we may have eugenics by the back door in the name of health through screens, treatments and therapies.

Other sociologists have raised concerns about potential eugenic outcomes due to prenatal screening for devalued traits (e.g. disabilities) (Shakespeare 1995), or the enhancement of humans through embryo genetic manipulation (Steinberg 1997). Rothman (1995) focuses specifically on associations between eugenic ideologies and prenatal diagnosis. She asks: how do we keep populations healthy (1995: 8)? Screen out the potentially unhealthy; this she argues is the basic eugenic principle. Selectively reproduce the fit and eliminate the unfit. That is how prenatal diagnosis works; potentially unhealthy newborns are screened out as fetuses, aborted and the health of the newborn population is supposed to be improved. But where, she asks, do we draw the line? If Down's syndrome, why not Turner's; if blindness why not severe myopia, if deafness why not hard of hearing (Rothman 1995: 8)? In our quest for the perfect baby through reproductive genetics where do we draw the line? Needless to say as Rothman highlights what is implicit in this use of prenatal technologies is the ideology that some genes are better than others, that some lives should be preserved while others prevented. Even when the logic of individual choice is emphasised – as it is in contemporary practices of prenatal screening and diagnosis – the focus is still on producing a normal child and preventing disability (Kerr 2004).

The aim of this chapter is not to explore the potentially eugenic nature of reproductive genetics this has already been recounted on numerous occasions (Rothman 1986, 1995). The aim of this chapter is twofold; to explore the gendering of good and bad genes and to look at who (men or women) takes responsibility for the production of these so-called 'good' or 'bad' genes. In using these terms I acknowledge that they are problematic – what is perceived as good or bad is obviously a subjective and heavily loaded process. Furthermore, genes for good and bad behaviours and health are continually 'discovered' only to be lost at a later date making any kind of fixing of genetics impossible (Conrad 1994). By good genes I am referring loosely here to the production of 'normal' blood screening results and the passing on of what was perceived by respondents to be good genetics, that is, good health, looks, physical appearance. Bad genetics refers to illness and other perceived problems identified with the fetus through prenatal screening. As others have argued men have often been associated with the production of so-called 'good genes'. Men's seeds and semen are viewed as the 'sparks', the 'life givers' of pregnancy while women are arguably perceived as caretakers of the fetus (Rothman 1986). However, should women receive 'risky' prenatal screening results or diagnosis then they are often viewed by society as bad reproducers, with ineffective wombs accused of producing children with faulty or defective genes (Finger 1990; Ettorre 2000).

Drawing on data from the study, this chapter will highlight the gendered association of so-called 'good' and 'bad' genes in prenatal screening. As the findings of the study show, men are often concerned with the establishment of good genetic connections between themselves and the fetus. They tend to focus on passing on their own positive genetic attributes to the fetus. Women, on the other hand often take responsibility for the health of the fetus and for positive or 'risky' screening results. However, the chapter will move on to show that maternal associations or responsibility for the production of potentially poor genes (through risky screening results) is not straightforward but is complexly mediated by a number of other factors including ethnicity, screening type and views on disability (Reed 2009a). Furthermore, men in some cases also take responsibility for potential genetic problems, particularly when they too have to be screened (as may already be the case in screening for inherited blood disorders). Thus as will be argued, the gendering of good and bad genes is complex and contradictory, both challenging and reinforcing traditional gender roles.

Reproduction and the gendering of genetic responsibility

Drawing on the views of experts in the field of prenatal screening and diagnosis Elizabeth Ettorre (2002: 88) argues that reproductive genetics constructs the idea that genetic capital, pedigree (i.e. pure breeding) and ultimately social fitness can be ranked. In biological terms genetic capital is related to the labour processes needed for survival. Ettorre (2002) argues that genetic capital should be perceived as that physical capital which functions to establish one's genetic identity and status in society (p. 82). According to her, the ranking of genetic capital is carried out in already unequal social contexts in which gender and disability are devalued. Women's bodies are caught between those ranked according to their pure breeding potential and those ranked according to discursive systems of inequality (i.e. class race gender). What emerges from this according to Ettorre (2002) is the view that on the one hand there are those women who are good reproducers with sound wombs who are capable of breeding well and with healthy genes. Such women have 'good' genetic capital. They should reproduce children and make babies. On the other hand there are women who are bad reproducers with problematic wombs and poor-quality genes (Finger 1990; Ettorre 2002). These women have the potential to reproduce genetic mistakes or give birth to children with illness or disability. Their bodies are flawed and they should not be encouraged to reproduce. Ettorre (2002) argues that this is an unintended social consequence of reproductive genetics creating divisions between good and bad reproducing bodies.

According to Ettorre (2002) therefore women appear to be divided into good and bad reproducers according to their genetic potential. However, when we look at this potential across the gender divide and its impact on the gendered nature of genetic responsibility the debates become more complex and contradictory. As Rapp (2000) has argued, across divides of class, ethnicity, nationality and religion many individuals hold mothers responsible for fetal quality and health. Each parent is allocated a 50 per cent contribution to the hereditary materials of a fetus during the moment of conception. As Rothman puts it, children are viewed as 'half his, half hers' (1995: 3). However, Rapp argues that the egalitarian nature of genetic (or blood) contributions are held in tension with a second, enduring and non-egalitarian idea, the highly gendered notion of maternal responsibility (Rapp 2000). Therefore, it appears that while women and men make equal contribution to the genetic make-up of the fetus women are the ones that take responsibility for the production of a quality fetus (Reed 2009a).

A number of studies in both the UK and US have highlighted the ways in which women take responsibility for fetal health. During pregnancy women are disciplined through the discourse of biomedicine, through texts and health professionals to comply with guidelines for healthy pregnancy behaviour (Marshall and Woollett 2000; Rapp 2000). Women are made aware of the correlations between certain lifestyle factors such as smoking or drinking and low birth weight, and the effects that some behaviours can have on genetic or chromosomal anomalies. For example, it is well recognized that one of the key factors in producing a child with Down's syndrome is the age of the mother with the risk being higher after the maternal age of 35 (Rose 1987; Ettorre 2002). Thus women are made aware that their choice to get pregnant over 35 increases the risk (NHS Down's Syndrome Prevention 2008). Furthermore, diet and folic acid intake are known to affect the prevalence of spina bifida and other neural tube defects. Therefore, women are advised by health professionals both pre-conception and during the first 12 weeks of pregnancy to take folic acid. This is because it is linked to reducing the risk of problems developing with the baby's spine and brain (NHS Down's Syndrome Prevention 2008).

Potential fathers do not carry a fetus and are therefore exempt from such pressures as pregnant women. In many cultures men are pictured as providing the creative seed or spark which causes the pregnancy without taking on any behavioural obligations which affect its outcome (Rapp 2000). The subtle distinction therefore is already in place, men have a direct and positive genetic contribution through creating a life. It is up to women and their wombs to nurture those genes to ensure they reach their full potential. As argued earlier, Rothman (1986) locates these gender differences between genetics and responsibility in patriarchal thought. At the core of patriarchy is the recognition of paternity as the idea that children grow out of men's seeds. Through patriarchy a distinction is marked between 'seed' and 'soil' – between paternity and maternity (Rothman 1986). Men and their 'seed' are viewed as the potential 'life giver'; women on the other hand represent the soil, the vessel for men's seed (genes). According to Rothman (1995) this distinction is then upheld in the scientific field of genetics whereby genes and DNA are routinely associated with paternal ties whilst maternal ties continue to be associated with nurture and childrearing. As other authors have pointed out, however, in the reproductive context pregnant women are viewed as the receptacle for theirs and their future offspring's genes (Ettorre 2000). When it comes to prenatal screening therefore, studies have tended to show that women take responsibility when screening detects a genetic condition or chromosomal anomaly (Rothman 1986; Rapp 2000; Reed 2009a).

Dragonas (2001) illustrates this well in her study on Greek women with 'risky' prenatal screening results and invitations to undergo amniocentesis. She found that these pregnant women had a sense of responsibility and accountability for a potential 'faulty embryo' and hence they experienced shame and guilt. She argues that shame was readily available to pregnant women because pregnancy affects them in a more primordial, direct fashion than it does men. Ettorre (2002) further reinforces this argument. She argues that women bear the burden of reproduction per se as well as the production of valued, non-disabled offspring. Women also bear the responsibility for children who are not so perfect. Landsman (1998) suggests that we live in an age of flawless babies and as a result, mothers of disabled children are seen as 'defective merchandise', their pregnant bodies as embodiments of motherhood have failed to follow the culturally appropriate trajectory (Ettorre 2002: 86).

Existing research therefore has focused on the ways in which reproductive genetics has the unintended consequence of identifying women as either 'good' or 'bad' reproducers depending on their genetic potential. This literature also shows how women take the major responsibility for fetal health, for producing a genetically acceptable child. Men on the other hand appear to be interested in the more positive manifestations of their own genes in reproduction. Drawing on data from the study this chapter will explore two interrelated issues: the gendered association of so-called 'good' and 'bad' genes and the subsequent gendering of genetic responsibility. The first section will focus on men and the positive manifestations of the paternal 'seed', subsequent sections will explore gender roles and 'risky' screening results. As will be argued in the conclusion, the gendering of good and bad genes is complex, depending on screening type and men's role. As will be shown this is also further mediated by other issues such as ethnicity and views on disability (Reed 2009a). Overall the chapter reinforces the argument that has been made throughout this book so far – that men's roles in screening both challenge and reinforce a traditional gender division of labour.

Routine screening and the establishment of 'good' genes

This section will focus on exploring the gendered nature of so-called 'good genes'. In particular, it will focus on the ways in which men in the study were often most interested in positive manifestations of their genetic input to the fetus. This was articulated by men through discussions over the inheritance of particular physical traits passed from them to the fetus and through the establishment of normal screening results. This can be placed in contrast to women's views. Throughout the study women were less interested in routine genetic connections or whether the baby might look like them and more concerned about the health of the fetus. Data from this study therefore certainly appear to resonate with Rothman's (1986) argument surrounding distinctions made between the seed and soil, between positive paternal genetic contributions and women's roles as nurturers and fetal containers.

The importance of positive paternal manifestations of genetics has already been touched on in Chapter 3; men within the study took an interest in what they viewed as a routine or positive manifestation of their genes. For example, as shown earlier one respondent Alan wanted to know whether the baby would share his blood type. As will be explored in this section, men were also specifically interested in positive physical attributes that the baby might inherit from them. This contrasted with women's views as demonstrated in the account below from Emma who was in the second trimester of pregnancy:

> All he kept going on about was whether the baby would take after him or me. To be honest, all I really cared about was whether it was ok. I wished he stopped going on about it all the time.
>
> (Emma, 22, Nanny)

Men were particularly interested here in the routine passing on of their 'good genes' to the baby. Many men within the study did not focus on whether they would pass on 'bad' genes such as hereditary illness. They wanted to know whether their offspring might have their physical prowess, be tall, be good at sport, etc. This is reflected in the quote below from Nick whose partner Sarah was in the second trimester of pregnancy:

> Well, you do wonder how your genes are passed on, will he look like me, have the same colour eyes. Will he be good at sport? I hope so, once we knew we were having a boy, I sort of hoped he be good at sport, especially football. I'd love that! I still play now and I hope it's something it I'll be able to do with him, once he arrives.
>
> (Nick, 32, School teacher)

Men therefore were more interested in visible physical manifestations of their genes rather than the general health of the fetus. There were also clearly gender differences in the views about the production of 'normal' screening results. As highlighted before the idea of 'good' or 'normal' genes is problematic for a number of reasons. Finger (1990) argues that the concept of 'normal' rose with industrialism. She argues that prior to industrialisation words like 'normal' and 'defective' had only been used to refer to 'objects'. Through the process of industrialisation these terms began to be used to refer to people. 'Normal' is used broadly in prenatal screening to describe prenatal screening results which indicate a low risk of fetal anomaly or to show the absence of women as carriers of genetic traits such as sickle cell. As argued earlier, women were less concerned about the physical attributes the baby might inherit from them and were more interested in receiving 'normal' screening results indicating a healthy fetus. This was particularly the case around results for routine screening. As Kerry who was in the second trimester of pregnancy states: 'We were so relieved when everything came back normal. I just wanted to know that everything was ok so I could start to enjoy this pregnancy' (Kerry, 29, Housewife).

In several cases women situated their own fears about the health of the fetus in stark contrast to their male partners. This can be seen in the account from Suzie below who was in the second trimester of pregnancy:

> It's, I don't think that he had as many concerns as I had. I've thought to myself what if, what if the baby was born with such and such, but I don't think he has as much. Or maybe he has and we've not discussed it between us, I don't know. Erm, but, you just, there wasn't anything really, we just, I think it be honest, we just don't like to think about what if the baby's not perfect, we'd rather come to that if it happens.
>
> (Suzie, 34, Housewife)

When female respondents received 'normal' screening results, they did not reflect on how this was associated with their own good genetic capital. They did not congratulate themselves as 'good' reproducers; rather, they related this to the importance of taking maternal responsibility. When their partner's screening test was normal, however, men tended to ruminate on their own genetic contribution to the health of the fetus. This is reflected in the quote from Bill below whose partner Kerry was in the second trimester of pregnancy:

> Well when they told us everything was looking ok, it was a relief. We both felt happy. You sort of feel like you have something to do with that, I mean, I know it's her that's pregnant but you know, my genes are in there somewhere!
>
> (Bill, 37, Electrician)

Occasionally, men did also talk about their own 'rude health' and how that might manifest itself in the fetus. This can be seen in the account from John below whose partner Christine was in the third trimester of pregnancy. He saw himself as being in good health and hoped that the baby would inherit that good health from him. When the midwife used a fetal heart rate monitor (see Chapter 3) to indicate a strong fetal heartbeat, John related this to himself:

> Well, I've always been fairly healthy, pretty robust actually. I sort of hope the baby will take after me like that. … When we go to see the midwife she puts that thing on my wife's tummy and says, "ahh its got a good strong heartbeat that one". Makes me feel proud, like I've had something to do with it!
>
> (John, 37, Currently unemployed)

Men within this study wanted to see how their 'good' genes were passed onto the fetus. They often wanted to know how the baby might inherit their sporting prowess or might look like them. This tends to reinforce existing arguments about the gendered nature of genetics as articulated by authors such as Rothman (1986). When it came to receiving normal blood screening results men also liked to reflect on the impact of their own genetic contributions. Women on the other hand were less interested in how screening results reflected their own biological make-up. They tended to focus on the health of the fetus, articulating a clear sense of maternal responsibility.

Women, men and the identification of 'bad' genes

So far this chapter has focused on exploring the gendered nature of so-called 'good' genes. As shown in relation to screening, both men and women were relieved when routine screening proved 'normal'. However, men in particular used these results as a time to reflect on their own genetic input into the health of the fetus. Within the following sections, I want to explore whether this was still the case when women had received 'risky' or positive screening results. In these instances the chapter will focus on gender and responsibility for potential genetic problems. A complex picture will be highlighted. This section will show that when it came to blood screening for inherited blood disorders men did not blame women for 'poor' genes but often took equal responsibility because they also participated in screening. However, when it came to high-risk screening results for other conditions where diagnostic testing took place solely on women, such as amniocentesis, then men took less genetic responsibility. One respondent Rosie gave birth to two children who both had been diagnosed with microcephaly. As will be shown in this case, a clear gendering of 'bad' genes is illuminated along with a reinforcement of maternal responsibility. The section will conclude by arguing that the gendering of so-called 'bad genes' and subsequent articulations of genetic responsibility are often complex and conflicted (Reed 2009a).

Gender equality and positive screening for inherited blood disorders

The notion that there are simply 'good' and 'bad' genes as shown earlier is somewhat complex and contradictory. Take for example, the case of sickle cell anaemia. This condition as argued earlier can result in disability and early death. In contemporary society therefore the associated gene is viewed as problematic, as something that should be identified where possible prenatally and the illness prevented. However, its high incidence in regions where malaria was prevalent during the 1950s led British biologist Anthony Allison to consider the possibility that it was associated with selective advantage. He discovered that having the sickle cell trait conferred resistance to malaria. In environments where malaria is prevalent carriers are more likely to survive childhood and reproduce so this variant has been perserved by natural selection despite its associated disadvantages

(Allison 1954; see Pilnick 2002). Despite this potentially positive aspect of the trait, negative associations of this genetic trait are currently manifest in British society. Screening to prevent children being born with blood disorders is a crucial part of prenatal care in the UK. Furthermore, recent studies have reinforced the argument about the eugenicist potential of screening programmes which in many places continue to be selectively targeted towards certain ethnic groups (Dyson 1999).

Several female respondents, as already discussed, received positive results for haemoglobinopathy screening. Subsequently men were often recruited for screening in order to determine the likelihood of the fetus being identified as having a blood disorder. The female respondents (as articulated elsewhere) who tested positive for sickle cell and thalassaemia were all very pragmatic about their positive result (Reed 2009a, 2011b). This can be seen in the account from Jameela, an African student who was in the third trimester of her first pregnancy. She had received a positive test for sickle cell anaemia and her partner Tunde was subsequently tested:

> No, I didn't feel as bad about it (the positive test) because he had to be tested too. My test was positive and his test was negative, which we sort of knew beforehand. It was no big deal and he was happy to be tested anyway.
>
> (Jameela, 37, Student accountant)

As mentioned earlier, when women tested positive for the sickle cell or thalassaemia trait, men were also tested. In these instances, women did not appear to blame themselves for the production of 'bad' genes or shoulder the responsibility for fetal health in this context. Responsibility for the genetic health of the fetus tended to be mostly shared with male partners. This is highlighted in the account from Jameela's partner Tunde, a doctor, who was tested for sickle cell and received normal results. As the quote below shows, he was more than happy to do this:

> Why would I put her through the pain and anxiety of amniocentesis when I could have a simple blood test to rule out any problems? There isn't a history of sickle cell in my family and I wasn't too worried but even so, I'm the father so I should be involved.
>
> (Tunde, 37, Psychiatrist)

The shared nature of genetic responsibility in this context was articulated by other respondents. For example, Pinky, in the second trimester of pregnancy had tested positive for the thalassaemia trait. Just like Jameela, Pinky also discussed the ways in which it was taken for granted that her partner would be screened and that they would share responsibility. This can be seen in her account below.

> Yeah, I mean it's your baby you want everything to be alright and we worried, but he was with me all the way and never hesitated about being tested himself. I mean, he's the dad isn't he?
>
> (Pinky, 30, Bank clerk)

In this context women did not seem to blame themselves for the production of 'poor' or faulty genes. They seemed to share this responsibility with their husbands and partners. This can be seen in the accounts from Pinky and her husband. Pinky's husband Bihar reinforced her comments about sharing responsibility and was happy to be screened:

> Well, it's our baby so it's our responsibility. She might be carrying it but I'm the dad so I need to take responsibility too. She had the thalassaemia gene so I had to be tested. It was frightening because what happened if we were both positive? We were both really worried but fortunately it was ok in the end.
>
> (Bihar, 31, Shop owner)

The respondents who tested positive for sickle cell or thalassaemia were largely Black African and South Asian. However, there was one female respondent Sarah who tested positive and who was ethnically white. Sarah was in the second trimester of her first pregnancy. Although she did not take quite such a pragmatic view about screening as the other respondents, again Sarah did not appear to blame herself for the production of so-called 'poor' genes, rather she emphasised the importance of her partner's involvement:

> Well, I was worried sick when I received the positive result. They (genetic counsellors) kept telling me the test was border-line and not to worry because he (partner) was white and it was unlikely he would be a carrier. But I was so glad he was tested, it made me feel it wasn't all down to me and that with his genes we had another shot at a healthy baby. He was great too, very laid back and supportive.
>
> (Sarah, 33, School teacher)

There was only one male respondent, Paul, whose partner Flo received a border-line test for thalassaemia, and who did not get screened. This couple decided jointly that he would not be tested. The reason given for this related to the fact that her test was only border-line, and her partner was ethnically white, and so they felt there was little chance of him being a carrier. As Paul's quote shows: 'Well we didn't see much point in me being tested as the potential for me having it was low. I would have been happy to but Flo felt there was no need' (Paul, 31, Self-employed).

What was interesting in this context was the lack of blame attached to women for the production of so-called 'poor genes'. Men did not appear to blame women for positive screening results but took part in screening themselves in order to ensure the health of the fetus. Of course the lack of male refusal to be screened, coupled with the fact that all male respondents in the study had negative screening results, does limit the generalisability of the findings of this study (Reed 2009a). Male refusal to be screened or a male positive result could result in women experiencing a heightened sense of maternal responsibility for the production of sickle cell or thalassaemia trait as has been shown by research on thalassaemia screening in India (Chattopadhyay 2006). However, in this study where men were screened, their direct participation did seem to indicate a shared sense of responsibility between women and men. Women did not appear to be 'blamed' in this context for the production of problematic genetic traits which may result in ill health of the fetus. Rather responsibility was shared. Furthermore, both men and women tended to take a particularly pragmatic approach to screening, particularly ethnically Black African and Asian respondents who knew family and friends who had experience of these conditions. However, when it came to the identification of 'risky' screening results for conditions like Down's syndrome, respondents' views were more complex.

Ultrasound, diagnostic testing and female accountability

In the UK the number of babies being born with Down's syndrome has increased since the introduction of prenatal screening from 717 in 1989 the year the technology was introduced to 749 in 2006 (BBC News 2008). As argued earlier this relates perhaps to the greater public awareness and positive image of Down's syndrome in the UK (Down's Syndrome Association 2011). It may also relate to the increase of women who are becoming pregnant and giving birth who are aged over 35. In such cases perhaps a longed for baby with illness or disability maybe deemed better than no baby at all (Shakespeare 2008). Screening for Down's syndrome was often a very emotive issue in the context of this study; while most women decided to participate, four couples opted not to have the screening or further testing.[1] This perhaps illustrates the complex and contradictory nature of views on issues such as Down's screening. Finger (1990) illustrates these contradictions well, drawing on her own experiences as a disabled woman and as a new mother of a potentially disabled child. Reflecting on her own experience she shows that on the one hand people often espouse positive views on the preservation of babies with disabilities whilst still wishing our own children to be born 'normal' (Finger 1990). Certainly couples in this study were often conflicted in their views on this issue. Some respondents did extensive research on conditions such as Down's syndrome, and decided not to opt for screening. These respondents emphasised the lack of certainty in the technology itself, further reinforcing some of the arguments made by Rothman (1998) about where do we place the limits to genetic screening. This view was prevalent in both women and men's accounts. This can be seen below in the account from Liz who was in the third trimester of pregnancy:

> I think there was quite a lot of information that the midwife gave me (on screening), plus you've had your first appointment. I guess as well … you just pick up information don't you, about Down's and Spina Bifida and things. Then there's things like Cerebal Palsy which they don't test for,

> which is a disease, and you know. I just find it a bit odd that you know, they kind of fixate on Down's and Spina Bifida when there are other things that could potentially go wrong that you don't get a test for at all. So it just seemed you know, a bit of an odd thing to have to worry about.
>
> (Liz, 32, University researcher)

As argued earlier, in Chapters 1 and 2 many respondents were more concerned about screening for chromosomal anomalies than they were screening for inherited blood disorders. Blood disorders were often viewed by respondents as less serious and tended to be associated with black and minority ethnic populations.[2] Therefore many ethically white respondents did not think that they were at risk of being genetic carriers. Furthermore, respondents tended to view conditions such as Down's syndrome as occurring randomly across the population, and as being a potentially severe disability. This is articulated by Emma:

> Erm, a bit more scared. Because the other tests that they do, they're more rare (blood disorders), less chance of having them in pregnancy and they can be solved quite easily. Obviously with Down's syndrome there's no cure to that, you just have to make the best possible life you can. So, yeah I'm a little bit worried. Not so much because of my age, because I'm not in that risk category (age 35 or above). I think it's about 21 to 25 isn't it? That's the best time to have a child. Erm so that gives me better odds, but still, I do know someone who was young and had a Down's syndrome child, erm. So I'm a little bit more anxious kind of thing, because they are very severe obviously. Spina bifida as an illness and Down's syndrome as a disability, so yeah, they're a bit more scary these ones (tests).
>
> (Emma, 22, Nanny)

Couples' attitudes to screening for Down's syndrome were often quite conflicted, so too were gender roles and responsibilities during this screening and diagnostic testing. In cases where serum screening had indicated a high-risk factor for Down's and spina bifida women's accounts demonstrated a palpable sense of genetic responsibility while men seemed to take less responsibility. Maternal responsibility in these cases was directly embodied as women's bodies, and women's DNA became the targets of diagnostic testing such as amniocentesis (Reed 2009a). This is articulated by Flo. She had received 'risky' test indicators for Down's syndrome for both her first and second pregnancies. Her quote below highlights her feelings of maternal responsibility towards this:

> I felt there was a sense of responsibility, because yeah, the mother's carrying the baby. … Me and Paul (her partner) are equals and he was with me every step of the way, but it's my pregnancy and so when I had to have the amniocentesis I did feel like it was down to me more.
>
> (Flo, 35, Self-employed)

The gender dynamics that were played out between men and women regarding routine screening for Down's syndrome were complex. While men often took part in decision-making about women's routine participation in screening (as was highlighted in Chapter 4), when a test was presented as high risk, women seemed to assume responsibility. This was directly related by women to their bodies, their genes and to their material existence. This can be seen in the quote from Linda who was in the third trimester of pregnancy:

> The first pregnancy I had a high result come back on the spina bifida one and it was just awful … I was due to see the midwife the next week or something, but it was just really, you know, it made both of us really worry and stuff. But I felt particularly anxious, you know because it's my body. But then, I had the scan and everything was fine.
>
> (Linda, 30, Childminder)

It is important to stress that within this study, although several respondents received high-risk results for Down's and spina bifida screening, the results of further screening or diagnostic testing came back as normal. As already stated in the introduction this book can therefore make no claims about the nature of men's roles when these conditions are actually diagnosed. When diagnostic testing was an issue or where women had to participate in ultrasound again for conditions such as spina bifida, women seemed to take more genetic responsibility. However, there were some examples of men taking more genetic responsibility. For example, Ben, whose partner Suzie was pregnant with her second baby (their first baby together), discussed the ways in which having a brother with Down's syndrome affected his feelings of responsibility during screening:

> Well, with Down's syndrome we gave it a lot of thought. I have an older brother with Down's syndrome and so I thought about it a lot and wondered whether that might be in the family somehow. This was my responsibility because it's my family. We decided in the end not to have the test because of my experiences. It wasn't just me but her as well. She's pretty strong minded, so if she hadn't agreed with me it wouldn't have affected anything, she would have made her own decision, but luckily, we felt the same.
>
> (Ben, 34, Customer support technician)

The importance of kinship and genetic family ties is something that will be explored in more detail in the next chapter. However, through Ben's account, we can see that there are occasions where men also take genetic associations and responsibility regarding screening for chromosomal anomalies such as Down's syndrome.

Respondents' views on screening and diagnostic testing were often quite complex perhaps mimicking broader complex and contradictory views espoused by society and the medical profession on this particular type of disability. When it came to gender roles for this type of screening these varied according to whether screening was routine or high risk. As shown in the previous chapter respondents tended to share decision-making over whether to opt for routine screening. However, in contrast to screening for blood disorders, when it came to diagnostic testing for Down's syndrome women appear to take more responsibility for the health of the fetus. This supports earlier literature on women, shame and maternal responsibility for the production of poor screening results (Dragonas 2001). However, there was some evidence that men took genetic responsibility in the case of Down's syndrome screening based on personal experience as shown in Ben's account. However, no woman's pregnancy within this study resulted in a diagnosis of Down's syndrome following amniocentesis therefore it is hard to fully explore the full gendered nature of genetic responsibility. In the last section of this chapter, however, the case of one couple will be explored where two children with learning difficulties had been born as a result of a potential maternal inheritance of a neurological disorder. As will be articulated, in this particular case we can see a clear gendered association of 'poor or faulty' genes.

Microcephaly: a case of bad female genes?

There was one couple within the study where female responsibility for the production of so-called 'bad' or defective 'genes' was specifically emphasised, and that was in the case of Rosie and Pete. Rosie was in the second trimester of her fifth pregnancy. Her children shared several different fathers. Two of her children had been born with microcephaly, a condition which her current pregnancy was also being monitored for. She was also being monitored for gestational diabetes which was identified as a recurring problem in her family (to be explored in the following chapter). Rosie's partner Pete was supportive during her pregnancy and screening (although he did not always attend appointments) but ultimately it was Rosie who identified microcephaly as a result of her 'faulty genes'. This section will focus on the experiences of Rosie and her partner in detail in order to explore the ways in which women appear to take ultimate responsibility when genetic problems are identified with the fetus.

Microcephaly is not something that this study originally sought to explore as the original aim was to focus on blood screening for inherited blood disorders or chromosomal anomalies. However, microcephaly was an issue that was raised with regard to two respondents Rosie and Pete. The identification of this condition among two of Rosie's existing children meant that she took part in extra ultrasound scans throughout her current pregnancy to make sure that the baby's brain was developing properly. Microcephaly is a neurological condition sometimes referred as small head syndrome. This is where the circumference of the head is smaller than normal because the brain has not developed properly or has stopped growing. As stated earlier microcephaly can be present at birth or it may develop in the first few years of life. It is most often caused by genetic abnormalities that interfere with the growth of the cerebral cortex during the early months of fetal development. It is often associated with Down's syndrome, chromosomal syndromes and neurometabolic syndromes. Depending on the severity of the accompanying syndrome, children with microcephaly may have learning difficulties, delayed motor functions and speech, facial distortions, dwarfism or short stature, hyperactivity, seizures, difficulties with coordination and balance, and other brain or neurological abnormalities. In some cases children with this condition will have normal intelligence and a head that will grow bigger, but they will track below the normal growth curves for head circumference (NINDS 2011). Rosie's existing children who had been diagnosed with microcephaly showed signs of some learning difficulties as a result.

During the interview Rosie immediately talks about the presence of her so-called 'faulty genes'. She does this initially to identify her concerns about screening for Down's and spina bifida. She relates this to her prior experience of giving birth to children with learning difficulties:

INTERVIEWER: Yeah. And did you feel differently about the two sets of tests, because the first lot they test for things like HIV, anaemia, thalassaemia, and the second lot are for Down's syndrome. Did you feel differently about the two?

ROSIE: Well I wasn't so concerned about the first one (first set of tests) because I'd never have got anything (like those conditions in the past), but the second lot (for chromosomal anomalies), I wondered if them faulty genes got in the way, but it (fetus) were alright.

(Rosie, 27, Housewife)

Most of the interview with Rosie related to her experiences and concerns over microcephaly. After discussing attitudes to routine screening for Down's syndrome Rosie went on to talk mostly about her experiences with microcephaly. Rosie discusses the need to participate in extra ultrasound scans during pregnancy to monitor her baby's development:

> Because I've got two children that are fine and I've got two children that have got these small heads aren't so fine, so they keep an eye on this baby. I've got one scan on Thursday to see if it's growing alright and then if not then I'm back to going every week.
>
> (Rosie, 27, Housewife)

Within the context of this study Rosie and Pete were interviewed together. It is through this joint interview and their conversations about microcephaly that we see a clear gendering of genetic responsibility. During the interview Pete articulated some concern over her current pregnancy and over whether the fetus might develop microcephaly. However, he made it clear that this problem was related to Rosie and that she did not want him involved:

> Erm, yeah, I think, Rosie obviously knows what's happening really and I'm not as worried as I was with John (previous child). I'm worried about the microcephaly business; I'm worried about this small head syndrome. I would be going to more (to appointments with her), but you (Rosie) don't seem to want me there too much anyway!
>
> (Pete, 31, Plasterer)

As the interview progressed Rosie talked more openly about her children being affected by microcephaly. Rosie took complete responsibility for her children developing this condition. Throughout her interview she talked frequently about how the problem with the children was her fault and related to her 'faulty genes':

ROSIE: Yes. Of course, Warren's (son) got problems, Claire's (daughter) not as bad, but the thing is could I cope with another child with all that because I've got two already. I've got two that are fine, it's just, like that, because it's my faulty gene and that's why it's gone on to my children.

INTERVIEWER: How do you know it's your gene?

ROSIE: They did my head and my head's size o' sixteen year olds. So my head is pretty small. When I were younger they never tested anything like that.

(Rosie, 27, Housewife)

What comes across during the interview with this couple is the way that Rosie identifies the 'bad genes' as coming directly from her whereas she sees her partner Pete as having 'good genes'. Rosie clearly views herself as someone with 'low' genetic capital whereas she ranks her partner with 'good' genetic capital. She was quick to reinforce his 'good' genetic potential throughout the interview. As she states: 'Because everything's (poor genes) on my side from having me children before, they tend to look into me and there's nowt (nothing) wrong with him' (Rosie, 27, Housewife).

Accounts from her partner Pete tended to reinforce Rosie's view. He talked about his own family and how there were no genetic problems within his family. He totally distanced himself from the production of these problematic genes: 'Well, I knew it wasn't in our family. There's nothing in our family except asthma and you can't test for that' (Pete, 31, Plasterer).

Through the accounts of both Rosie and Pete therefore we see a clear gendering of 'good' and 'bad' genes and subsequently of genetic responsibility. One final issue raised by Rosie and Pete's interview was the role of health professionals in the construction of women as either 'good' or 'bad' reproducers. Towards the end of the interview Rosie discussed the role of the midwives and other medical professionals and their views on her particular case. She felt that they held quite stereotyped and negative views towards her, as a mother of five, with several children who had learning difficulties. This can be seen in her account below:

> They were perfectly nice to me but I get the impression that they thought, here we go again. Why doesn't she just pack it in. you know, they look at me with me five kids, not all have got the same dads and some of em with problems and you know they make assumptions.
>
> (Rosie, 27, Housewife)

Accounts from this couple then highlighted the ultimate gendering of genetics. Rosie directly identifies and blames herself for the production of faulty genes. She took total responsibility for two of her children having the condition microcephaly whereas Pete was quick to distance himself from the production of bad genes. There may be an obvious material reality to this as two of her children had already developed the condition. Maternal inheritance therefore probably played a role in this context. However, the accounts shown here highlight the differences of maternal and paternal responsibility prevalent during the diagnosis of genetic conditions. This reinforces arguments made by others around women's sense of responsibility for the production of poor genes during screening (Dragonas 2001; Ettorre 2002). It again also reinforces Rothman's (1986) argument about the positive contributions of paternal seed. Furthermore, this case was the clearest illustration in this study of the ways in which women are ranked by the medical profession according to their genetic capital (Ettorre 2002).

Conclusion

This chapter has focused on the gendered associations of the so-called good and bad genes. It has also explored the issue of genetic responsibility. For example, who takes responsibility when screening produces 'normal' results and who takes responsibility when things go wrong? As has been shown, gender roles in this context are often complex and contradictory. When women receive good news about screening, both women and men are happy that their dream of having a 'normal' baby is kept intact. When 'normal' results are received, however, women tend to just exhibit relief. Men, however, while pleased that screening results were 'normal' also reflect on their genetic contribution to such normality thus reinforcing men's association with the production of so-called 'good' genes'. As shown through the accounts of both women and men, men often reflect on their passing on of 'good' genes through the baby inheriting their looks or sporting prowess, etc. This reinforces Rothman's (1986, 1998) argument about the importance of positive paternal contributions to the fetus.

However, as was also explored during this chapter, what happens when screening places women at increased risk of giving birth to a child with disabilities or illness? In these cases the gendering of good and bad genes and the gendered nature of genetic responsibility are indeed complex. Female respondents seemed to exhibit a strong sense of embodied responsibility for some positive screening results. In these cases, in support of earlier studies women did appear to blame themselves for the production of 'faulty genes' (Finger 1990; Ettorre 2000). This blame, however, was not extensive and did appear to be related to the type of screening in question and also to men's direct participation in screening. For example, when it came to positive carrier screening for inherited blood disorders men and women took fairly equal roles in the process. This was largely associated in this study with the fact that in most cases men were also subjected to screening.

When it came to screening for chromosomal anomalies such as Down's syndrome women, however, seemed to take more genetic responsibility than men. This supports the findings of earlier studies on women's experience of amniocentesis and the shame and responsibility due to the associated production of so-called 'defective genes' (Dragonas 2001). Within this study women's keener sense of genetic responsibility relates undoubtedly to the fact that women and women's bodies and blood are the ones directly subjected to screening and diagnostic testing. Men's material existence plays no direct part in this. It also relates perhaps to the often complex and contradictory views many lay people hold on the issue of disability particularly with conditions such as Down's syndrome. As argued earlier, couples often held very strong views on the issue of Down's syndrome screening and four couples decided not to opt for screening. However, respondents also tended to be more frightened about this particular type of screening. Anne Finger (1990) illustrates the complex views often held by people on the issue of pregnancy and disability in her book *Past Due*. Finger, a key advocate in the US disability rights and women's movement is also a physically disabled woman herself after having polio as a child. Despite this, after having a traumatic labour which had the potential to result in her own child developing disability or learning difficulties, Finger wills her own child to be 'alright' whilst acknowledging she will love him despite illness or disability:

> I understand that under capitalism, the concept of normalcy is used to reinforce the standardization necessary for industrial culture. That children are seen as possessions, commodities. While in my head it repeats like a chant: I don't want anything to be wrong with him, I don't want anything to be wrong with him, I don't want anything to be wrong with him. And that sits side by side with my knowledge that I will love him no matter what.
>
> (Finger 1990: 171–72)

It is important to note here that within the context of this particular study, although several respondents tested as positive or high risk for conditions, no one was diagnosed with any conditions, All respondents interviewed went on to have 'normal births'. The ability therefore to explore the gendered nature of genetic responsibility on diagnosis of this condition is therefore impossible.

There was one case in the study as shown, however, where the gendering of good and bad genes and the subsequent gendered nature of genetic responsibility was extremely clear. This was in the case of Rosie and Pete and the condition of microcephaly. Rosie had already given birth to two children with microcephaly and therefore had first-hand experience of the implications of raising children with learning difficulties. The diagnosis of this condition in two of Rosie's existing children led her to trace it directly to her own 'faulty genes'. As a result Rosie took full responsibility for the fact that two of her children had the condition and had learning disabilities as a result. Rosie's partner Pete was clear to distance himself from this process reinforcing the gendering of genetic responsibility. Within the antenatal clinic Rosie was made to feel like a 'bad' reproducer by health professionals for continuing to get pregnant and have children when she already knew there was a genetic problem. This then reinforces two issues. It reinforces the associations between women, reproduction and maternal responsibility as outlined by other authors (Rapp 2000; Reed 2009a). It also reinforces the argument put forward by Ettorre (2002) that women tend to be labelled through the discourse of biomedicine as either good or bad reproducers – an assessment which is partly based on whether women are deemed to have good or bad genetic capital. Furthermore, it reflects some of the issues explored earlier on the eugenic potential of screening as women appear perhaps to be subconsciously either discouraged or encouraged to reproduce depending on their genetic potential.

Overall, throughout the chapter the complex and often contradictory nature of gender and genetic responsibility has been explored. Again what appears to be highlighted here is a complex set of gender roles. On the one hand men do get involved and take responsibility for the production of both good and bad genes thus suggesting a shift away from traditional gender roles. On the other hand the extensive nature of maternal responsibility is never far from the surface. Within this study women still continue to take the ultimate responsibility when things go wrong with the pregnancy. In the next chapter the focus of the book will broaden out its focus purely on men and women to include an analysis of the roles of family and friends in screening.

6 Family, friends and heredity

Introduction

So far, this book has focused on an exploration of gender roles within screening. In particular it has focused on exploring the roles that men and women take in the process as partners and as potential parents. Within this chapter I want to move away from focusing specifically on men and women's roles to explore the roles of wider family and friends. While highlighting the specific importance of the roles played by partners and health professionals in women's pregnancy, a number of studies have highlighted the importance of friends and family. General studies on pregnancy have shown that friends and family can have an important role in a woman's pregnancy through offering practical and emotional support to women (and more recently men) as women progress throughout various stages of pregnancy (Dunn *et al.* 2003). At times friends and family may also influence decision-making over screening (Carroll *et al.* 2000). In recent years, studies on genetics have focused on the more direct role played by kinship and family history. Family genetic history is perceived to be a useful clinical tool used in order to assess an individual's risk of developing particular diseases, for example, colon or breast cancer (Yoon *et al.* 2002). Genetic testing including prenatal testing has come to form part of this family risk assessment. Women may be offered particular prenatal screening based on family history of disease. In turn, prenatal screening may throw up genetic traits which lead people to turn detective on their own family history. Furthermore, experience of kinship and disability may further impact on couples' decisions to opt for prenatal screening (Rapp 2000). The role of family in screening therefore can be significant in the context of prenatal screening.

In light of this, the aim of this chapter is to situate the gendered nature of prenatal screening in a broader social context. It will explore the importance of external factors such as family and friends on gender dynamics in prenatal screening. The chapter will begin with an exploration on the influence of friends. Throughout the study friends often influenced couples' decisions to opt for certain types of prenatal screening, particularly the use of technology not available free on the National Health Service such as nuchal fold screening.

Family also affected screening decisions and sometimes contributed to conflicts between men and women. Family influence in screening also has a more direct influence on genetics and gender roles (Rapp 2000). As will be explored, within the study respondents often had a general awareness of the role of family genetic history. At times this awareness of history affected attitudes towards prenatal screening, particularly in cases where family members suffered from various inherited disorders. Family history also had direct clinical implications when genetic links were identified, sought out and monitored. Overall, the chapter will emphasise the positive roles that family and friends can play in couples' experiences of prenatal screening-both indirectly through supporting women and their partners during screening and more directly through family history and inheritance. However, the chapter will also emphasise the ways in which male partners remain more important in advising and supporting women during pregnancy and screening than family and friends. Furthermore, family and friends sometimes lead to minor conflicts between couples and again tend to reinforce the gendered nature of genetic responsibility.

The Importance of family and friends

Studies on women and pregnancy have often highlighted the importance of both friends and family in supporting and advising women throughout the process. For example, in their research on socially disadvantaged women and smoking in pregnancy in Midwest USA, Dunn *et al.* (2003) emphasise the important roles of female confidantes. Their study demonstrates that pregnant women often identify a single, close female friend or relative who provides advice about pregnancy-related issues. In their study they found that confidantes were often more persuasive than women's partners on general pregnancy-related issues and at least as persuasive as partners on smoking-related issues. Confidantes in their study were most often mothers, with other significant relationships being sisters and friends. They tended to find that although confidantes were seen as less influential than doctors, they had more intimate and frequent contact with the expectant woman. This tended to highlight the importance of their influence. Overall their study points to the importance of recognising the roles of friends and relatives in pregnancy in informing and advising women.

Studies on other aspects of pregnancy have highlighted similar results. For example, Hollyer *et al.* (2002) conducted a study in the US on pregnant women's use of Complementary and Alternative Medicine (CAM) for pregnancy-related conditions such as nausea and vomiting. They showed that CAM was used by almost two-thirds of their respondents for nausea and vomiting in pregnancy. Most women within their study got information about CAM from their family and friends. Again therefore, the role of family and friends in information giving and advising women during pregnancy is emphasised. While most studies have focused on the role of family and friends in informing pregnant women, the role of friends and families is also emphasised in the newly emerging work on men as fathers-to-be. For example, Finnbogadottir *et al.* (2003) conducted a Swedish study on the experiences of first-time fathers. They found that during their partner's pregnancy men became part of a daddy's club, connecting and sharing experiences with other fathers.

General research on pregnancy therefore has highlighted the important roles of friends and family in advising pregnant women (and men) on a range of pregnancy-related issues. Studies on prenatal screening in particular, have also tended to emphasise the relatively important role of friends and family both as advisers and supporters of pregnant women. Carroll *et al.* (2000) for example conducted a study on women's experiences of maternal serum screening (MSS) in Ontario, Canada. In their study they found that pregnant women turned to their social support networks for help in making decisions about testing. This included partners, family and friends. The degree of involvement of women's partners ranged from couples who had extensive discussions about the risks and benefits of MSS to women who independently decided whether or not to have a screening test. Other family members, particularly women's mothers, had a great influence on their decisions. Women's shared experiences and stories from friends affected their decisions on whether to have MSS. In particular, shared bad experiences, often in the context of false-positive results had a profound effect on how women viewed MSS.

When it comes to diagnostic testing such as amniocentesis, studies have often shown that family influence and support can be conflicted. For example, in Rapp's (2000) study on amniocentesis in the US, she found that family support for amniocentesis could be both positive and negative. On the one hand, there were cases in her study whereby family could be incredibly supportive offering to help look after a child born with disabilities. On other occasions respondents' families could be judgemental of their decisions to participate in diagnostic testing and in some instances in selective abortion. This occasionally led to women lying to family if a problem was detected with the fetus. Some respondents felt that in such cases they would tell family that they had suffered a miscarriage rather than the fact that they had decided to abort a fetus due to the diagnosis of anomalies. The influence of family therefore can work both ways in the realm of prenatal screening and diagnosis.

While most studies on pregnancy and prenatal screening identify a role, albeit a conflicting one for both friends and families, other studies have urged caution to the importance of the role of family and friends either as supporters or advisers of pregnant women. For example Learman *et al.* (2003) conducted a study in the US on attitudes towards prenatal genetic testing for Down's syndrome. Their focus was to explore these attitudes across a diverse range of ethnic groups. In their study all groups reported highest levels of influence by partner or husband and health professionals and lowest by friends and religious leaders, with family members intermediate. Therefore they argue that perhaps the role of friend and family as supporters and advisors should not be overestimated in assessing influences on pregnant women.

Existing studies therefore tend to show some disagreement over the extent and nature of the roles played by family and friends as both supporters and advisers of women undergoing prenatal screening and testing. Aside from support and advice, however, there is another more direct role played by family in this context. That is the role of family history in determining genetic risks. The notion of genetic inheritance has grasped the imagination of those with a family history of various diseases for example breast or colon cancer. The role of inheritance in disease potential is firmly established (Fox-Keller 1992). Both the mass-media and doctor–patient relationship tend to amplify people's emphasis on biological kinship and the realisation that family and kin pass on disease. In light of this an extensive family history is at present the key tool used by modern medicine to estimate an individual's risk of disease. Acquiring a family history requires detailed information from an individual about their relative's ages, medical problems, relationships ancestry and ethnicity (Finkler *et al.* 2003). Such risk assessment through family history may then lead to genetic testing to further identify risk (Yoon *et al.* 2002).

Inheritance plays an important role in the pre-prenatal and prenatal realm. For example, fragile X syndrome and cystic fibrosis are both inherited conditions which can be screened for both pre- and during pregnancy (Genome 2007). Family genetic history can also play an important role in prenatal blood screening and diagnosis. For example, sickle cell anaemia and thalassaemia major are autosomal recessive conditions where individuals who inherit a deleterious gene from both parents develop the disease (Atkin, Ahmad and Anionwu 1998). As argued earlier, inheritance of an affected gene from both parents leads to a one-in-four chance of the fetus developing either one of these disorders, whilst inheritance of one abnormal gene results in a healthy carrier (NHS Antenatal and Newborn Screening Programme 2008). Therefore family history (alongside ethnicity in this case) may have a direct role in identifying 'at risk' women. For other conditions that are screened for prenatally the role of inheritance is less well known. For example, Down's syndrome is not a directly inherited condition. However, there are a small number of cases where a woman's chance of giving birth to more than one baby with Down's syndrome is increased. This occurs when Down's syndrome develops due to chromosomal translocations (this accounts for around 4 per cent of cases). This process involves the transfer of part of one chromosome to another and may reflect an abnormal chromosome arrangement in one of the parents. If this is the case the chance of a further child having Down's syndrome is significantly increased. Family history and genetic testing may therefore prove useful cases such as these (NHS Evidence 2011a).

Drawing on data from the study this chapter will explore the indirect and direct roles played by friends and families in prenatal screening. The first part of the chapter will focus on assessing the roles of family and friends, as advisers and supporters of pregnant women during screening. As will be shown family and friends have some influence on screening decision-making and can be a great support not only to women, but also to men and couples. However, family can also lead to conflict among couples themselves. Furthermore men's roles as supporters and advisers during their partners' pregnancy, tends to surpass those of family and friends. The chapter will move on to explore the more direct role of family through family history and inheritance. The chapter will ask what role does family play in women and men's attitudes towards, and experiences of prenatal screening. In what ways are men and women aware of family history? How does a positive screening result affect respondents' sense of kinship? As will be shown, both male and female respondents have a reasonable interest in issues of family history and how it may potentially impact on the health of the fetus. However, while men do show an interest in family history and in some cases do detective work on the family past, the major responsibility for family history still rests on women's shoulders.

Women, men and the role of friends

In support of the findings of earlier studies on pregnancy, unsurprisingly perhaps, friends did play a role in women's accounts within this study. As shown earlier, in Chapter 1, women actually often found that they drew on the experiences and advice of friends during pregnancy. This is articulated in the quote below from Katarina a Czech respondent who was at the end of her first trimester of pregnancy:

> Well my friends have been really important sort of generally during the pregnancy, I mean they have already been through stuff so I can ask their advice. I mean, not necessarily about screening but more about pregnancy and about how I'm feeling.
>
> (Katarina, 28, Self-employed)

Along with general friendship influence during pregnancy, women also talked about the roles that friends played specifically in relation to screening. This is reflected in the account below from Emily who was in the second trimester of pregnancy:

INTERVIEWER: So you talked to people who have been through it (pregnancy and screening)?

EMILY: Yes, I definitely talked to some of my friends about it, and my family. Whether going for tests and things was helpful, and what decisions would you make from that, and so, yes, I had some discussions with other people

(Emily, 30, Health professional)

Sometimes women's friends had a direct influence on women's screening choices. This is demonstrated in the account below from Eleanor who was in the third trimester of pregnancy. Eleanor had opted to have a nuchal fold scan during her pregnancy. She had heard about the nuchal fold scan not from her midwife but from friends. As already stated at the time of data collection nuchal fold scans in the context of this study were only available in private hospitals. Sometimes midwives would tell women about the scan including which private hospitals offered it. However, often they did not. In these cases women tended to hear about the scan from other sources including friends:

INTERVIEWER: Do you mind me asking about why you got the nuchal fold scan?
ELEANOR: … Yeah. It was because I was over 30 I think, but also a friend of mine who, well I've got friends in London. They get it (scan) free on the National Health Service down there and we don't here. … I just in my last pregnancy I had the nuchal scan as well and I think I just wanted to know. Because my friends had had one as reassurance so we thought we'd have one.

(Eleanor, 34, Director of a family company)

Most women within the study, however, felt that while they might discuss screening options with friends that ultimately they made their own decision about whether or not to opt for screening. This is highlighted in the quote below from Rebecca who was in the second trimester of pregnancy:

> Well, some of my friends did decide not to have the tests, you know, for Down's syndrome and that. It didn't affect me though I made up my own mind about the tests in the end.
>
> (Rebecca, 36, Housewife)

Some women in particular felt that although they discussed testing with friends that ultimately decision-making was between themselves and their partners. Again this reinforces the findings of studies such as Learman *et al.* (2003) that place the importance of male partners above friends and family during women's pregnancy. This can be seen in the account below from Kerry who was in the second trimester of pregnancy:

> No, it was very much the two of us. I mean we've got, as I say this time round, more friends who are pregnant and two of them have decided not to have any testing. And we've decided to have everything. Yeah, just different people. And they're all a lot older than me as well.
>
> (Kerry, 29, Housewife)

Similarly another respondent, Joanne, felt that decision-making over screening was a private matter involving only pregnant women and their male partners. She related this in particular to the implications of bringing up a child with disabilities for women and men as a couple.

INTERVIEWER: What are the things that have influenced your decision to have blood screening? Did you talk to any friends about it or your family or do you think it was just you as a couple that makes decisions?

JOANNE: I think it is very private, yes I do because that final decision you would have to live with it. I don't think either of us have thought about it too much but particularly when you are talking about Down's. Down's children can live really quite normal lives but is up to individual couples themselves to decide how that would impact on them.

(Joanne, 35, Nurse)

As the accounts from women show, friends did play a role in women's pregnancies and their discussions around screening decision-making. However, most women reinforced the findings of existing studies by highlighting the importance of ultimate decision-making with their male partners (Learman *et al.* 2003).

Along with discussions on the influence of female friends on decision-making, both women and men also discussed the significance of friendships with other couples. Women and men felt that their relationships with other couples who had gone through or were going though similar experiences in pregnancy and screening could be useful. This is articulated in the quote from Lucy who was in the second trimester of pregnancy: 'Quite a few of our friends have had babies before us and you do pick up quite a lot (of information) from them' (Lucy, 35, Hospital doctor). Accounts from men tended to reinforce this view as the quote from Liz's partner Brendan shows:

> We've got three friends in the last year that have been in the same situation as us, and I don't think there's any better sort of advice than from people who know you. We asked our friends a lot of questions.
>
> (Brendan, 33, Travel agent)

Some women within the study drew comparisons on men's involvement in pregnancy and screening across their own friendship groups For example Brendan's partner Liz discussed the ways in which you could see trends towards men's greater involvement. She looked across at other friends who were having or had recently had babies and discussed the ways in which men's roles differed now to the ones they held in the past:

> But I think men are becoming more involved generally in the process. Certainly all of our friends, the fathers-to-be are very actively involved in pregnancy and screening and all the rest of it. So, I think, yeah, it's up to the individual but I think more men are taking a more active role, or have been more able to; it's more socially acceptable for men to take an active role in pregnancy.
>
> (Liz, 32, University researcher)

Several men in the study also talked specifically about the importance of their own male friends in being supportive and offering advice on pregnancy and screening. As Jan's partner Alan states:

> Yeah, sometimes it was helpful to talk to the lads; you know the ones who have already been through it. Fortunately I had a few mates that had had babies and that helped.
>
> (Alan, 40, Plumber)

This perhaps supports the findings of earlier studies such as Finnbogadottir *et al.* (2003) which highlighted the importance for men of friendships with other fathers, their own father and fathers-to-be. For men within the study friends sometimes had a much more important and direct role. One respondent in the study, Brendan, discussed the impact of growing up with a friend who had Down's syndrome. He highlighted the ways in which this friendship shaped his views on screening and disability during his partner's pregnancy:

> Yeah, well I was saying when I was growing up, I had a good friend who had Down's syndrome and until I was sort of old enough to really get my head round it, he was my mate, he was my friend. And I grew up with the kid. Until you're six or seven years old and you realise there's something wrong, and you're like why isn't he doing what we're doing? You know what I mean. And then it's explained to you that he has something and all that sort of stuff … and this has shaped the way I think about disability now.
>
> (Brendan, 33, Travel agent)

Data from this study did show that friends played some role in informing women and men's experiences of prenatal screening. The role of friends varied from directly influencing women's decision-making over which tests to opt for to offering general advice about pregnancy. Couples' friendships and male friendships also played some part in supporting and advising couples over screening. However, as argued earlier while worthy of consideration the role of friends was not central in respondents' accounts. What appears clear in respondents' accounts here is the importance in particular of men's roles in screening and the primacy of couple decision-making. When it comes to the role of the family, however, this had more significance for both women and men.

Family influence in prenatal screening

Family of both female and male respondents played a role in informing their attitudes to screening and decision-making. Family of course may mean different things within different cultures and to different people within those cultures, and not all of these meanings will be based on blood ties on which genetics is based (Pilnick 2002). In order to distinguish these differences Pilnick (2002) draws on Richards' (1996) threefold conceptualisation of kinship. Richards suggests the use of three terms–kinship, close family and household. Kin represents the wider extended family such as aunts, uncles and grandparents. Close family are kin with whom we may currently co-reside, for example, parents, siblings, etc. Household may be more complex due to issues of divorce or remarriage, and so may include relationships which may or may not be based on blood ties (Pilnick 2002). Family influence in the context of this study on screening referred mostly to close family and wider kin including parents and siblings. As with other studies on pregnancy women talked in particular about the importance of female relatives such as mothers and sisters who offered both emotional and practical support during pregnancy (Dunn *et al.* 2003). Couples also discussed the role of their 'parents' more generally in screening. While family was mostly perceived to be supportive, there were cases within the study where family led to conflict between women and men. There were also examples of couples and women in particular conflicting with extended family over diagnostic testing. Within the study therefore the role of family was both one of conflict and support.

Mother knows best

Mothers and sisters were undoubtedly two of the most important sources of support and advice for women in this study. Many women emphasised a close relationship with their mother who was often secondary only to their partners during pregnancy and child-rearing. As Eleanor states: 'Er, my Mum. I'm very close to my Mum; she does a lot with my other little boy. So yeah, my Mum, nobody else really. Really my Mum and my partner' (Eleanor, 34, Director of family company). Sisters also played an important role here. Sisters were often particularly important to women when they were also pregnant or had already been pregnant and had children. This is shown in the quote from Jan below who was at the end of the first trimester:

> Well, it was good because my sister got pregnant around the same time as me. It was really nice we both knew what each other were going through and could help one another out. We did talk about the tests as well. I wouldn't say she influenced me particularly but it certainly helped to talk it through with someone else.
>
> (Jan, 32, Hairdresser)

One respondent, Suzie, actually talked about the ways in which both family and friends were important to her during pregnancy and screening. In fact, contrary to others studies which place family as being of limited significance in comparison to the role of health professionals (Learman *et al.* 2003), this respondent talked about the ways in which she trusted family and friends' advice above that given by health professionals during pregnancy. As Suzie states:

> Yeah, as it turns out, well no, my sister hasn't (experienced pregnancy), but most of my friends have, have got children, and obviously I talked to me mum because she's done it! (laughs) But yeah, I mean, I probably do talk to family members and friends sort of more than a health

> professional, in a silly way. Because it's life experience that you want to know about, you know, what happened with them (when they were experiencing pregnancy/screening). A midwife can tell you what happens in sort of a hospital situation, with strangers, but I like to find what other people have done (about screening), that I know.
>
> (Suzie, 34, Housewife)

While mothers and sisters often gave women emotional support during pregnancy and screening decision-making, they also offered practical support. For example, when men could not attend screening appointments due to work commitments it was often women's mothers or sisters that they took with them. As Christine, who was in the third trimester of pregnancy, states: 'If he couldn't go I'd take me mum. She was always happy to be involved' (Christine, 34, IT consultant).

This was a common occurrence for many women. Women often ended up taking mothers or sisters along to screening appointments. This was because antenatal screening appointments tended to take place during the day. As already explored in Chapter 2, men often could not get time off work to be involved. In some cases men looked after women's existing children while women were attending appointments. As the quote from Rosie highlights:

> The kids come home from school and it (appointment) often clashes with that. He sometimes looks after them (kids) and so I either end up just going on me own or getting me sister or getting me mum to come with me. But it depends on what time the appointment is.
>
> (Rosie, 27, Housewife)

The majority of men found the input by mothers-in-law really useful in this context. They felt bad when they could not attend antenatal appointments due to work commitments, and were glad when mother-in-laws or other female relatives could step into the breach in their absence. This is reflected in the account below from Rebecca's partner Bill.

> Actually her mum did offer to go with her to her antenatal appointments if I couldn't go, and to be honest I were glad of that you know because I don't want her (partner) to be on her own.
>
> (Bill, 37, Electrician)

However, this was also used in some cases by men to suggest that mother-in-laws were too involved in their partners and their lives. The stereotype of the interfering mother-in-law was never far from the surface on these occasions. In some cases therefore women's mothers' involvement led to conflicts between women and men. This can be seen in the account from Jan's partner Alan below:

> To be honest, I think her mum would be in the delivery room if she could! She is so involved. Every time she's (wife) had an appointment to see the midwife my wife's been running to her mums to talk about it you know. They are always together and its baby this baby that, does my head in!
>
> (Alan, 40, Plumber)

Men also sometimes suggested that their pregnant partners actually preferred going with their female relatives to antenatal clinic rather than going with men themselves. As Rosie's partner Pete states: 'I would be going to more, but you don't seem to want me there too much anyway! You go with your sister and your Mum more than me don't you?' (Pete, 31, Plasterer). However, there was also suggestion that this type of male attitude was a bit of an excuse. There was also some suggestion during interviews with some couples that men used women's female support networks as a way to absolve them of having to participate in prenatal appointments. This can be been in Rosie's retort: 'Yeah that's your excuse (laughs)!' (Rosie, 27, Housewife).

Women, men and the role of family

While women talked most candidly about the importance of female relatives, couples also discussed the role of their parents. One respondent Eleanor spoke about involving her parents in everything to do with the pregnancy but also added that things had changed significantly since 'their day':

> We're a close family so I do like to involve me mum and dad on what's going on. Although, I didn't talk to them too much about the tests, they couldn't really understand as it was over 30 years since my mum had been expecting.
>
> (Eleanor, 34, Director of a family company)

Another respondent Christine found her parents really helpful during her pregnancy and screening because they were both health professionals themselves:

INTERVIEWER: Ok. And were your friends or family involved in those sorts of things? Did you talk to anybody else about them (tests), or was it just your partner?

CHRISTINE: I think, erm, yeah, with the things like the Down's. Because my parents are both in the health service so I did speak to them.

(Christine, 34, IT consultant)

Again though, while couples did acknowledge the role of their parents in advising and listening to them in discussions over screening, on the whole respondents often suggested that parents had very little impact on their actual decision-making around testing. This is articulated in the accounts from Liz and Brendan below:

BRENDAN: It all influences, everything does, no matter what.
LIZ: Yeah, but I wouldn't have said that us asking our parents, they didn't tell us not to have the tests or anything, it was nothing like that.

(Liz, 32, University researcher and Brendan, 33, Travel agent)

Some couples lived away from their parents, with quite significant geographical distance between them. As a result again they often felt that family and kin had a limited impact on the pregnancy and their decisions over screening. This can be seen in the accounts below from Kylie and Sean:

KYLIE: Just trying to think, my family is abroad, your family is in Ireland.
SEAN: Yes they (family) have been fairly removed, they are not particularly involved, I think because they are older and everything is different now. So there is that sort of level that they are that much removed. They are also in a different country and it's another level of removal.

(Kylie, 28, Nurse)

This particular couple were the only couple to explicitly discuss the influence of religion on their attitudes towards pregnancy and screening. This couple identified themselves as Christian. In the absence of biological kin in the area, they identified their church as their family. They found religion to be a very influential force on their attitudes towards screening, and more generally as a source of support during pregnancy. As Sean states:

> So it would have been a lot harder to talk to them (family) about screening and also we don't … we tend not to. … We didn't ask our parents on that (screening) because it was a very black and white issue for us. It wasn't the kind of an issue we needed some help to think it through. Although our church community. … it is just like family an extended family. So in a sense our family is physically distant but it also quite a close knit (religious) family in Sheffield.
>
> (Sean, 30, Self-employed)

The importance of religion in informing health beliefs has been highlighted in a number of previous studies (Reed 2003). The importance of religion in the context of attitudes towards prenatal screening has also been highlighted in the context of prenatal screening and diagnostic testing (Rapp 1998). Within this study religion was not something central to most respondents' accounts. However, for this particular couple religion provided an important source of advice and support. Some respondents therefore found support from sources other than family, when family was emotionally or physically distant. Other couples did not involve family in screening decision-making until after the 12-week pregnancy milestone, when a viable pregnancy was established through the 12-week scan. This can be seen in the account from Zoe: 'Well, we did involve family but only after I'd had my 12 week scan. By that stage I'd already had some of the tests anyway so there wasn't much to discuss really' (Zoe, 31, Museums officer).

In her study Rapp (2000) found that many women and their supporters make fine distinctions between relatives, deciding in whom they can confide about decisions on testing and when. For example, in her study she found that sometimes couples queried whether members of extended family could handle the issues raised by screening and testing psychologically. At other times for her respondents testing became a political issue for family. Couples were unsure at times as to whether wider family would approve of diagnostic testing and selective abortion (Rapp 2000). Within the context of this study on screening, family were mostly involved, but couples decided when and how much involvement they had. Also in the absence of family, couples drew on other forms of support. Despite the overall influence of family, the role of male partners and the decision-making that went on between couples was still of paramount importance.

Conflicting relationships, the role of extended family

As argued earlier, in her study on amniocentesis Rapp (2000) identified kinship as both a positive and negative experience for pregnant women and their partners. Family could be a great source of support to women offering to help look after a disabled child as a result of a positive diagnosis. It could also be negative. For example some women in her study did not tell relatives about testing because they felt that they would disprove. One respondent in particular said that she might lie to relatives and say that she'd had a miscarriage rather than a selective abortion as a result of a positive amniocentesis result. In this study, one of the respondents, Flo, received a risky maternal serum screening result for both of her pregnancies. She went on to have an amniocentesis in both cases. Both pregnancies resulted in the birth of children without disability or illness. However, she talks about the role of her extended family upon being faced with risky screening results and opting to have diagnostic testing. She identified in-laws in this context as both positive and negative. She has a supportive experience when she talks things through with her sister-in-law.

> I spoke to my sister and my sister-in-law, and my sister-in-law was probably more understanding about ultimately what decision I take, if the test was positive. My sister was, she was, I think she was probably quite surprised about my decision, but that's alright. But my sister-in-law and her husband, who has worked with people with learning disabilities for years they completely understood the decision, because of their personal experience.
>
> (Flo, 35, Self-employed)

Flo's experience here highlights the positive support of extended family through discussions with her sister-in-law. However, the same respondent also had a very negative experience during her interactions with her mother-in-law over the same issues.

INTERVIEWER: Did you talk to your mother-in-law?

FLO: She just rambled on about what she would do. Whereas I, the reason I don't discuss things is because I just need time to make my own mind up and think about things, and she was just talking about, regurgitating the same information which doesn't help at all. And the second time she knew nothing about it because I preferred it that way.

(Flo, 35, Self-employed)

The conflicting role of in-laws on women's health and health choices is something that has been explored by existing studies on gender and health often leading to a negative impact on women's health (Reed 2003). Certainly within this current study, the role of in-laws is perceived to be both positive and negative. This again highlights the complex and often contradictory roles of family as advisers and supporters during prenatal screening. In the next section the more direct influence of family on men and women's experiences of screening will be explored through focusing on issues of family history and genetics.

Family history and genetics

As argued earlier, family history is now perceived to be an important tool in assessing an individual's chance of developing disease from colon cancer to breast and ovarian cancer. Family and kin connections are framed in terms of genetic inheritance from parents, grandparents and other relatives. The increased use of family history in this context has led some to argue that there has been a medicalisation of kinship (Finkler *et al.* 2003). The medicalisation of family and kinship takes family beyond the realm of love and choice to the fixed and immutable realm of genetics. Family history may be used in primary care settings in order to predict an individual's risk of disease and to identify whether genetic testing should if appropriate be offered. Given the media hype around the role of family history in assessing disease risk, people have begun to turn detective exploring family history in the context of specific genes and illnesses as is the case for the BRCA1 gene and breast and ovarian cancers (Hallowell 1999).

A number of authors have identified difficulties in the use of family history in the clinical context. For example, discrepancies often exist between the uses of family history by lay people compared to the Mendelanian explanations of inheritance favoured by medical professionals. In discussing family genetic histories for example, patients may include non-blood relatives, or exclude blood relatives on the basis of their own interpretations (Pilnick 1996). Furthermore as discussed earlier in Chapter 3, the issue of physical likeness between family members is also of key importance in lay understandings of genetics. Individuals may perceive themselves to be at an increased risk of the inheritance of certain diseases as looking like someone often leads people to believe that they have inherited the same genes. Emotional closeness or distance to a relative may also be seen as an indicator of risk (Hall *et al.* 2007). This can make it difficult for clinicians attempting to assess the role of family history in an individual's disease risk.

Family genetic history when used in the medical realm often serves several functions. It may locate someone as being 'sick' even though they are actually symptomless. Furthermore, while family history places a person's risk of disease beyond their own control, genetic testing, including prenatal testing may offer individuals some means of control (Finkler *et al.* 2003). If no one in the family past or present has suffered from a disease, they too maybe protected. However, much genetic testing comes with no guarantees of whether a person will develop an illness. It offers risk assessment (Finkler *et al.* 2003). Family history may be used by clinicians in prenatal screening to determine someone's risk of carrying a fetus with a particular condition. For example, prenatal blood screening is used to identify inherited conditions as in the case of haemoglobinopathy screening for sickle cell and thalassaemia. These conditions are directly autosomal recessively inherited disorders and clinicians may use family history along with ethnic background in order to screen people who are deemed most at risk. Although not a directly inherited condition, family history may also be useful in the detection of Down's syndrome, as argued at the start of this chapter, in cases where chromosome translocations have led to the condition (NHS Evidence 2011a).

The aim of this section is to explore the importance of family history in respondents' accounts. Both female and male respondents did acknowledge at some level the potential role that heredity may play in influencing fetal and child health. There were cases where this became particularly important to respondents. This was often when certain conditions had been identified in other family members and subsequent monitoring of pregnancy was required, or where respondents had existing siblings with disabilities. There were also cases within the study where couples actually turned detective on potential family history to see how that might affect the health of their unborn baby. Furthermore, family history was also of key importance for women who tested positive for sickle cell or thalassaemia. In these cases kinship and ethnicity led women to develop certain practical attitudes towards screening.

Family history and pregnancy

Respondents within this study were asked a series of questions about family history. They were asked whether they were aware of any health problems in their family that might affect the health of their baby. They were also asked whether they had explored their family history for hereditary illness. The response from Emma below in the second trimester of pregnancy was a fairly common one:

> Yeah, so I've glanced in to it (hereditary illness). I haven't researched it deeply because I've never needed to. If something ran in the family then yeah I would look in to it more, but because there isn't really, I've only glanced at it.
>
> (Emma, 22, Nanny)

Other respondents' comments such as Rebecca's below reinforced this view: 'Yeah we have sort of thought about it, you know what the baby might inherit but to be honest there isn't much in either of our families to worry about' (Rebecca, 36, Housewife). There were times, however, when although women did not think they were likely to be carrying a baby with genetic problems, women did nonetheless think about the impact of their own family history on the health of the baby and on the baby's future. This was articulated in the account below from Chelsea, who was in the third trimester of pregnancy:

> Sometimes I do think about family illness and how that might be passed on. You know, there's a lot of heart problems and diabetes that runs in my family and sometimes I do wonder you know, will the baby have any of those. You do wonder sometimes whether you do the right thing by having kids.
>
> (Chelsea, 25, Care worker)

There were also cases where women's close relatives had been diagnosed with specific illnesses. In these cases women often did not know whether these illnesses were inherited or not. This again caused women to think about their baby and the implications that their own family history might have on the baby's future. This is highlighted in the quote from Trish:

> Well, actually my sister's depressed, well not just depressed but manic depressive you know. She's been ill off and on for years. I've heard that there's a gene for that, and sometimes I wonder.
>
> (Trish, 38, Academic)

Many women in the study were aware that their own genetic family history may have implications for the health of the fetus and also for the baby's future life. As will be shown in the next section, this was more pronounced in some cases where family history was used to detect or monitor certain conditions in pregnancy.

Detecting and monitoring family connections

There were cases where potentially inherited conditions during pregnancy had been identified among respondents' relatives. These genetic connections were then factored into the monitoring of respondents' current pregnancies. This was the case with Rosie, whose experience of children with microcephaly was discussed in the previous chapter. Microcephaly is a neurological disorder which has multiple causes, one of which is genetic. Rosie actually identified a genetic link with herself and her children. However, she did not discuss the correlation of her 'faulty gene' with other wider family members. She did, however, discuss at length a genetic link for gestational diabetes. Clinical research has indicated that diabetes can result from a multifactorial mode of inheritance where the fetus is more susceptible to metabolic teratogens (Van Allen and Myhre 1991). This can lead to fetal anomaly. In the case of this respondent, her sister had experienced gestational diabetes and had lost a child during pregnancy. As a result Rosie was also tested regularly for the condition.

ROSIE: Well before, my sister, when they first (tested her for diabetes), she thought everything were going to be fine but they didn't realise until it were too late, she actually had it (gestational diabetes). They did a post mortem on the baby and realised that she had a problem, and she ended up being diabetic, so they keep a close eye on me for that … Because my sister's diabetic I have to have like an extra test to see if I was diabetic or anything like that

INTERVIEWER: During your pregnancy?

ROSIE: Yes, because my sister's child died and they didn't realise she were diabetic. So all through my pregnancy they keep an eye on me and that's my test tomorrow (for diabetes). Last time it come back fine, but this time, I feel my blood sugars funny, I have to have Lucozade and chocolate with me, so I don't know what will happen.

(Rosie, 27, Housewife)

Rosie's case highlights the importance ascribed to family history in the prenatal clinic. In her case it was used to monitor her potential to develop gestational diabetes. There were other examples within the study whereby respondents had grown up with disabled siblings. This then affected their attitudes to screening and to bringing up a child with a disability. This was the case with Suzie's partner who had a brother with Down's syndrome. This in turn affected his feelings towards screening.

> Well, because his brother was disabled, he felt really strongly about it. No testing no way. Because he knew what its like, being close to someone with a disability. He always knew, no matter what we'd keep in it.
>
> (Suzie, 34, Housewife)

In her study on amniocentesis Rapp (2000) discusses the ways in which the consciousness of disability is formulated and shaped by a capricious sense of family history, and by the memories of kinship through which that history is constructed. Some women and men have had extensive experiences with disabled children, and told detailed stories of growing up with affected siblings. This sense of family history and experience of kinship and disability is evident in accounts from Suzie and Ben in this study.

Some respondents with 'risky' screening results for Down's syndrome such as Flo reflected on the potential influence of family history. Although both of Flo's pregnancies turned out 'normal', she did ruminate on the possible genetic connections with family resulting in risky screening results:

> Because it happened in both pregnancies you do start to think, does this run in the family? But as far as I know no one else has experienced this. Anyway, I had an amniocentesis and both babies were ok.
>
> (Flo, 35, Self-employed)

Within the study there were also respondents who turned detective on their family history. As Innes (2003) argues investigation or detection is a complex form of sense making, a way of seeking out unsuspected networks of connection and worlds assembled out of unforeseen arrangements of things (Austrin and Farnsworth 2005). Some respondents took this detective approach to unearth genetic problems within the family. They wanted to search their own history for genetic conditions which might influence the genetic health of their baby. An example of this was Emma's partner Jo who had grown up without his biological father. When Emma found out she was pregnant, he went off to trace his genetic history. Unfortunately Jo could not be interviewed as he was overseas with the British army. However, Emma his partner talked at length about his detective work in to his genetic past:

> There's nothing genetically that runs in the family that we know of. The only problem that we do have is that we don't know his real Dad. He grew up with a different Dad, so he's actually gone round to his Nan's and asked her to have a word with his dad. She did go looking for him (his dad), and asked him whether there was anything in his history. So he (Jo) has kind of looked into it quite a lot, so, I know it sounds silly but we were just thinking we couldn't take that risk because you never know what's hereditary in other families. He might even be a carrier of something that hasn't developed yet.
>
> (Emma, 22, Nanny)

There were examples therefore in this study, of both men and women where family history seemed to matter. Family history was used in the prenatal clinic to assess risk and monitor existing pregnancies. Respondents themselves also reflected on family history and its roles in screening. In some cases they even turned detective to assess the impact of family history on the health of the fetus. This reinforces the argument that you cannot escape genetic family ties. As Finkler *et al.* (2003) articulates, family genetic history takes us beyond arguments of choice in terms of family and kinship relationships (Giddens 1991). The notion of choice is the antithesis to the role genetics plays in assessing the effect of family on our future and our offspring's future health. In turn advances in the new genetics themselves, for example in relation to new reproductive technologies are also re-shaping the way we think about and relate to ideas about kinship (Edwards *et al.* 1993). On the one hand we emphasise the importance of genetic connections through genetic screening, whilst creating families with no genetic ties through technologies such as IVF using egg donor on the other hand. The overall effects of the new genetics on family and kinship are therefore often complex and contradictory.

Positive screening results and heredity

In this final section of the chapter the role of family history in screening for directly inherited blood disorders such as sickle cell and thalassaemia will be explored. As argued earlier these are autosomal recessively inherited disorders (NHS Evidence 2011b). They are passed on from parents to children through unusual haemoglobin genes (Antenatal and Newborn Screening programme 2010). Inheritance patterns are often horizontal, for example a generation may be affected (several siblings of the same parents), but not their parents nor their own children. Parents and next-generation children will usually be carriers. In ascertaining someone's potential risk, ethnicity is often a guiding factor as argued earlier in the UK, the groups more at risk are those identifying as Black African and Black Caribbean. Thalassaemia is more common among Cypriots, South Asians and Chinese, but also occurs among white British and Black African and Black Caribbean people (Atkin, Ahmad and Anionwu 1998). Family history may also be used in the clinical setting in order to determine women at risk, for example, locating existing family members with blood disorders (Chattopadhyay 2006).

Couples within this study affected by positive screening results often had prior knowledge of the disease, or knew a friend or relative who was affected by it. Sometimes therefore family connections were obvious. At other times when being identified as either sickle or thalassaemia carriers, some couples looked back into their family history to see where this trait might have originated. This can be seen in Pinky's account below:

PINKY: Well, as soon as we found out there might be a problem it was obvious he should be tested. We discussed it a bit with our families, tried to find out where it (thalassaemia) might have come from, but yes, ultimately, we decided about it as a couple.

INTERVIEWER: Did you manage to trace the origins?

PINKY: Well, there was talk of one of my relatives in India, having blood problems but people were a bit funny about it.

INTERVIEWER: What do you mean?

PINKY: Well, they didn't want to talk about it really.

(Pinky, 30, Bank clerk)

Pinky tried to explore the role of family history in the context of her own positive screening result for thalassaemia but found her family were not forthcoming. This reluctance on the part of Pinky's relatives to trace the gene in this study is perhaps culturally rooted. Chattopadhay (2006) conducted a study on prevention campaigns for thalassaemia in Bengal India. She found that one of the most important reasons why such schemes fail is because of the deep-rooted cultural notions of blood, marriage, identity and personhood and kinship in Bengal society. Blood is so deeply valued in the Bengal kinship system that this genetic mutation is perceived to be corrupting the blood – and affects marriage potential and future lineage. Thus in some cases, attitudes against screening may be deeply culturally embedded. It is possible that Pinky's family's reluctance to discuss the underlying role of family history relates to this issue. However, the culturally embedded nature of screening decision-making was not fully explored by this respondent within the context of this study.

As discussed earlier, Jameela, an African student, who was in the third trimester of her first pregnancy was identified as a sickle cell carrier through screening. This was no surprise to Jameela. She knew that the 'gene' had come from her as she claimed there was no history of it in her partner Tundes' family. She identified the sickle trait from her own family background:

JAMEELA: Well, I kind of knew it would be a possibility as it's in my family. My aunt had a child with sickle cell and I know that further back then that it's in the family.

INTERVIEWER: What grandparents?

JAMEELA: I think great-grandparents. I'm not sure. All I know is that we have had a history of it and so it was no surprise.

(Jameela, 37, Student accountant)

Although not discussed explicitly by respondents in this study ethnicity perhaps also has a role here. Apart from one white respondent, Sarah, the women who tested positive for blood-related conditions were South Asian, African and Mauritian. Inherited blood conditions are more common among certain ethnic minority populations then they are among white North European communities. In her study Rapp (2000), found that ethnic minority women felt quite knowledgeable about these conditions because they often knew sufferers within their families and communities. This meant that women often knew how the condition was passed on genetically and thus took a more practical approach to screening (Reed 2009a).

The one ethnically white respondent Sarah who tested borderline positive for the thalassaemia trait had no idea about the role of family history in her case, although she identified it as relating perhaps to Mediterranean blood way back in her families past.

INTERVIEWER: Was there evidence of it in the family?

SARAH: God no! I had no idea where it came from? I know that it tends to be more common in Black and Asian people and some Europeans. I know that I do have some Mediterranean blood so I assume it's from there.

(Sarah, 33, School teacher)

Sarah's account perhaps points to the racialisation of inherited blood disorders. Racialisation here refers to the ways in which ethnicity becomes an isolated and predominant variable in the identification and treatment of certain diseases (Reed 2003; Ahmad and Bradby 2007), possibly resulting in the development of selective screening programmes and potentially racist service provision[1] (Dyson 1995; Atkin, Ahmad and Anionwu 1998). Within the study Sarah was perhaps the only thalassaemia carrier identified through screening who did not already know the role of her family history. For most screen-positive female respondents, the importance of family history in identifying an individual's risk was something which was taken for granted. As argued in the previous chapter, in terms of screening for blood disorders men were happy to share responsibility for screening. However, ultimately when it came to the role of family history in assessing fetal health, women took the major responsibility.

Conclusion

This chapter has focused not only on gender roles in screening but on the wider roles of friends and family. As shown in this chapter, women did draw on their discussions with friends on screening related issues. In some cases friends had a direct impact on decision-making where friends informed women about particular types of screening. On occasions men also drew on relationships with other fathers-to-be. This could be a source of support for men during their partners' pregnancy. Mostly however, both female and male respondents emphasised the importance of relationships not with individual friends but with other couples also experiencing pregnancy and screening. As argued in Chapter 1, sharing experiences with others who had gone through or who were going through the process was often helpful to both women and men within this study. However, despite the role of friends in this context what became clear is the ways in which couples mostly saw decision-making as a private matter between the two of them not to do with their wider social networks. Furthermore, in women's accounts male partners' roles in screening were viewed as being far more important than the roles played by friends. This again emphasises the overall importance of men's roles in screening. As articulated earlier, this is also consistent with the findings of some earlier studies (Learman *et al.* 2003).

Family was more important to both male and female respondents than friends were. Family offered support to couples on both an emotional and practical level. Women often felt that their female relatives were important, especially mothers and sisters. This is because mothers and sisters had often already been through pregnancy themselves and could offer advice and support (Dunn *et al.* 2003). In many cases this support was practical. Many women took their mothers or sisters along to their antenatal screening appointments, especially when men could not attend. Couples also found the support of wider family such as their parents invaluable, again in advising and offering emotional support during screening. As Rapp (2000) found within her study, the respondents also highlighted potential conflict during pregnancy and screening with wider family. There was at times conflict between men and women over the extent of mothers' involvement in their daughter's pregnancy; men sometimes felt that mothers were too involved. Mothers' involvement, however, in some cases was also used by men to limit their own involvement. There was also conflict at times between women and in-laws over screening and diagnostic testing. Overall though, family played a supportive role to women and men during screening.

As argued in the final section of the chapter, family also played a more direct role in the process through the impact of genetic family history. A number of studies have highlighted the importance of family history in mapping and preventing disease. In light of this, family history has been used to assess an individual's probability of developing certain diseases such as breast and colon cancer. This has led some to argue that there has been a medicalisation of kinship (Finkler *et al.* 2003). While Giddens (1991) has emphasised the importance of issues of 'choice' in marriage and family, the new genetics eschews this notion of choice and kinship. You may choose a life partner but you cannot choose your family history – genetic history is fixed in a way that belies choice. This is an interesting paradox given (as argued in Chapter 2) the discourse of choice that currently surrounds the emergence of the new genetics (Rose 2001).

Both male and female respondents were interested in family history and how this might affect the health of their unborn child. Family history was also important for some respondents whose genetic family history and existing experience of disability may have an effect on the fetus. Some respondents (see Emma's account), even played the role of 'genetic detective', exploring their own or their partner's family genetic history in order to contribute to an assessment of fetal health. Family history was even more central for those respondents who tested positive for the sickle cell or thalassaemia trait. In these cases family history was often already known and the family link to disease often already established. Both men and women took an interest in their family history and its role on the health of the fetus. However, as concluded in the previous chapter despite a shared interest it did seem that women took the ultimate responsibility for the impact of their genetic past on the health of the fetus. Again this perhaps reflects the material reality of pregnancy occurring in women's bodies. However, it also reinforces the gendered nature of genetic responsibility; although men's role in screening is increasing, women ultimately continue to take most responsibility for the health of the fetus even regarding the impact of family history. Having examined the impact of broader social relations of family and friends in this chapter the following chapter will open up this debate further. The final substantive chapter focuses not only on the gendered nature of screening, but will also examine the relationship between screening, social class and race and ethnicity. In the process the chapter aims to explore the transformative potential of such screening technology.

7 Transforming social divisions

Introduction

As Kerr (2004) argues, a number of authors have outlined the potential transformative nature of the new genetics for social relations. For example, the emphasis on individual 'choice' inherent in the application of many of these technologies has the potential to transform individual biology (Rose 2001). This suggests that people can to a degree choose their own genetic futures, potentially subverting and reinterpreting our existing social hierarchies. As Kerr (2004: 5) states, these issues have been developed on a broader scale by authors such as Beck (1993) and Giddens (1990) in the context of a risk society and reflexive modernity. According to Beck (1993) technologies manufacture risks which have questioned the actual project of modernity. The centrality of consumer choice and large-scale technological hazards prevalent within a high or radicalised modernity have potential to undermine existing forms of social stratification and in doing so foster new forms of social order based on 'dialogic democracy' (Giddens 1990, 1991, 1992; Kerr 2004: 5). In this context the new genetics are viewed by some as part of this potential to challenge existing forms of inequality and create new social relationships.

However, while some view these technologies as potentially transformative others paint a bleaker picture. Some authors argue that medical innovation such as the new genetics can both reinforce existing forms of inequality as well as create new forms of inequality or exclusion (Webster 2007). For example, as already discussed in Chapter 5, genetic screening may provide for better screening of genetic mutation and disorder but thereby works to stigmatise those who are already disabled (Webster 2007). Furthermore, some have argued that the new genetics may create new forms of inequality. Webster (2007) uses the example of genetic screening in certain work environments. He shows that in some contexts genetic screening has been used to determine whether workers have a susceptibility or specific resistance to particular toxins used in that context. However, rather than making these environments clean to accommodate all, those with the least susceptibility have been employed. He argues that if pre-employment testing for a range of susceptibilities were to become the norm those with higher levels of susceptibility could effectively become unemployable (Human Genetics Commission 2002) creating a new form of inequality based on an individual's *genetic* capital (Webster 2007: 91). As argued previously this may have negative potential for governments who may use this as a rationale to cease addressing structural inequalities in society through policy. Rather than changing society to meet the needs of people, people will be created to genetically fit society (Pilnick 2002).

In light of these debates, the aim of this final substantive chapter is to explore the potential of new technologies such as prenatal screening techniques to transform existing social relationships more broadly. In this context it will move away from focusing its exploration explicitly on gender roles. It will focus instead on the relationships between prenatal screening and other types of social stratification. This chapter will explore the transformative potential of prenatal screening focusing particularly on issue of social class, race and gender. Drawing on data from the study, along with a wider body of literature on inequality and screening, this chapter will argue that technologies such as prenatal screening do present some challenge to existing forms of inequality along the lines of class, race and gender. As will be shown, while some social divisions existed between respondents within the screening arena, these were not as pronounced as perhaps those demonstrated in existing studies. As argued throughout this book, along with gender roles, prenatal screening both challenges and reflects existing and new forms of inequality. The chapter will conclude by returning to debates over the extent that technologies themselves have the potential to transform social relationships based on gender, class or race and ethnicity or whether they merely reflect or reinforce existing social circumstances.

Social class, ethnicity and prenatal screening

When it comes to issues of social class, race and ethnicity and screening existing research has seldom focused on any transformative potential of technology. Rather it has tended to identify the prenatal arena as an arena where existing inequalities of class and race are reinforced. Existing studies on women and prenatal screening and diagnostic testing in the UK and US have tended to explore two key issues in this context: who has access to screening and who uses screening services. In exploring these issues inequalities in terms of both social class and race and ethnicity have been at the forefront. According to Rapp (1998) among the structural reasons for rejecting prenatal testing, class associated differences loom large. Regarding prenatal screening, Rapp (1994) argues that women's comfort with the 'scientific worldview' is bound to be affected by social class, suggesting: 'It is an axiom of genetic counselling that middle-class patients (disproportionately white) usually accept the test while poorer women (disproportionately from ethnic minority backgrounds) are more likely to refuse it' (Rapp 1994: 222). Several studies have supported this, for example, Kuppermann *et al.* (1996) found women 'who listed their own or their partners' occupation as "professional" or "student" ... were significantly more likely to undergo prenatal diagnosis than others who indicated that they or their partners were homemakers, unemployed, or employed in blue collar jobs, regardless of racial or ethnic group' (p. 680).

A number of other studies have found that issues of class and culture affected women's likelihood of opting for screening. For example, Babay (2004) found socioeconomic position, alongside religion and education were all likely to influence the acceptability of prenatal testing. Given these results, economic position and the patterns associated with economically deprived areas (ethnic diversity, religiosity, poor education facilities) should be understood as factors, amongst others, influencing comparatively low figures of prenatal care utilisation amongst ethnic minority groups (Delvaux *et al.* 2001). Rapp (1994) situates screening uptake within a web of social factors suggesting: 'The intersecting fault lines of class, race, ethnic and religious differences, sexual preferences, experiences with disabling conditions, and so forth' all influence patients' decisions, in turn affecting their access to prenatal screening (p. 229).

While studies have shown that issues of class and ethnicity affect women's use of prenatal screening and testing, they are also likely to affect a woman's chance of being offered prenatal screening. Rowe *et al.* (2008) found that ethnicity and social class significantly affected the likelihood of patients being offered ultrasound and amniocentesis screening for Down's syndrome. Women from the most deprived social groups were less likely to be offered screening than others. Asian women were also, 'significantly less likely to be offered screening compared with White women' (Rowe *et al.* 2008: 1247). A number of factors have been identified as reasons why these differences exist in use of and access to prenatal screening services. Cultural differences in pregnant women's attitudes towards screening and issues of disability and abortion, along with racial discrimination on the part of health professionals have been two of the most enduring reasons given. What is clear, however, according to Rapp (1998) is that generalisations about class and ethnicity affecting take-up of prenatal screening and testing services require further exploration.

She argues that for example in terms of social class, differences in use of and access to screening are not as straightforward as often presented. It is often assumed in existing studies that working class women are more likely to reject screening while middle class women uncritically accept it. In her research on amniocentesis in the US, she found that private patients (that is, middle class ones) usually did not go for genetic counselling (to learn about amniocentesis) unless they were already determined to have the test. She argued that these women are likely to have prior knowledge about it gleaned from books, friends and private doctors. According to Rapp (2000) these women tended not to schedule an appointment with a genetic counsellor and therefore women who refuse testing in this class are rarely counted. Furthermore, in her study many women from working–poor backgrounds, including African American and Hispanic women do accept the test. Their rates of acceptance and refusal as recorded in hospital records vary dramatically from facility to facility. Furthermore, although Rapp focuses mostly on women, she does acknowledge that the class and ethnic backgrounds of male partners also affect women's use of screening. Rapp (1998) concludes that the effects of class, race and ethnicity are far more complicated than often presented in existing screening research.

This chapter aims to explore issues relating to race, ethnicity and social class focusing on how they mediate women and men's experiences of prenatal screening. The chapter will be divided roughly into two parts. The first half of the chapter will explore the relationship between social class and prenatal screening and social class and gender roles. The chapter will take a multi-faceted approach to the concept of class, acknowledging the interrelated but at times separate influence of different aspects of class identity from economic to cultural. As stated in the introduction respondents' occupations were categorised broadly in line with The National Statistics Socio-Economic Classification system (NS-SEC).[1] Some differences in respondents' attitudes towards screening across class will be highlighted according to a variety of issues from socioeconomic position to access to cultural capital. However, the chapter will mostly show that the influence of social class was not as pronounced as often portrayed in existing literature. Furthermore, when it came to issues of gender within this study, class had a limited impact on gender roles in screening. The clearest correlation here between social class and screening was related to men's ability to take time off work in order to attend their partner's screening. On the whole though, involvement across classes was similar.

The second half of the chapter will focus on issues relating to race, ethnicity and screening. This was a difficult issue to explore given the small sample sizes of minority ethnic respondents[2] in the study. However, despite this limitation some interesting issues were observed. Respondents did identify some issues of discrimination in the screening clinic, yet there did not appear to be big differences in attitudes towards different types of screening as often portrayed in existing studies. Ethnicity did not seem to alter gender roles in specific ways except as argued in Chapter 5 during positive screening for inherited blood disorders. In these cases black and minority ethnic respondents tended to espouse more gender equitable roles then white[3] respondents. However, what was interesting in this study was the issue of 'whiteness' and screening for inherited blood disorders. Ethnically white respondents tended to 'racially' distance themselves from this screening during interviews further reinforcing existing arguments about the racialisation of certain illnesses. Before moving on to focus in detail on issues of ethnicity however, in the following section the focus of this chapter will be on issues relating to social class and screening.

Social class, health and prenatal screening

Class inequality has been a pre-occupation of sociologists since the classic contributions of Marx, Weber and Durkheim (Webster 2007). Through the advent and development of industrial capitalism social stratification by social class was defined and measured in terms of an individual's occupation, income and ownership of wealth/property and clear class gradients were shown (Webster 2007). The connections between health and social class inequality have also long been the focus of medical sociology. For example as Nettleton (1995) highlights, reports on the labouring classes produced in the mid nineteenth century revealed those that were poor experienced more disease than those that were rich. Social class formed an important focus in sociology and in particular in the sociology of health and illness during much of the twentieth century. In recent years some have argued for the demise or death of class reflecting the decay of strong occupational communities, fragmentation of the labour process and the decline of trade unions (Webster 2007). Furthermore, the deterioration of these sectors has been allied with the growth of the consumer market through credit. This has according to some flattened out social differences based on consumer goods and lifestyles. Rather than traditional forms of social class, some suggest that consumption markets have produced highly fluid status groupings. People then choose to buy into such groupings rather than being constrained by the old class hierarchies and conventions (Pakulski and Waters 1996). Furthermore, an increase in social mobility and opportunity for women in the labour market has transformed the ways in which gender and class have been related (Webster 2007).

While some have argued that class is dead. Many others such as Scott (2000) argue that social class continues to structure our lives even if it does so in ways less palpable than before. Furthermore, while some continue to espouse the material base of class formation (Goldthorpe 2004), others prefer to focus on class as a lived culture, not just an objective entity but concerned with identification, perception and feelings (Medhurst 2000). One of the most popular approaches to social class in recent years is that put forward by Bourdieu (1979); he suggests a model of class which is based on capital movements through social space (Skeggs 1997). The structure of this space is given by the distribution of various forms of capital including economic (e.g. income), cultural (e.g. education), social (e.g. capital generated through relationships) and symbolic capital (relates to the legitimation of capital)[4] (Skeggs 2001). This view of class allows for an understanding of how people have access to different amounts of capital and embody certain dispositions (Skeggs 2001). It shows that social class therefore in contemporary society is both complex and contested, mediated through time and space.

According to Webster (2007) the traditional manifestations of social class hierarchies may be less apparent in contemporary society. However, access to material resources through social networks remains central to people's life chances both in the Weberian sense with respect to social standing and in the biophysical sense with respect to health and longevity. In the context of health, studies have consistently shown that health status and behaviours continue to be mediated by issues of social class and ethnicity (Reed 2003). As argued earlier in the area of antenatal care, similar patterns have been reported

(Lazarus 1994; Rowe and Garcia 2003). Although the main focus of this study was on gender, women and men were sought from a range of socio-economic backgrounds (see section on sampling and recruitment in the introduction) in order to explore the impact of social class on women and men's views on screening, and on gender roles taken during screening. The chapter will draw loosely on Bourdieu's (1979) conceptualisation of class utilising the four types of capital outlined earlier – economic, social, cultural and symbolic. What will be highlighted throughout this section is that while social class did play some role in the accounts of the respondents, this was far less of an issue than first thought. Furthermore, while economic capital led to the biggest class differences in screening (especially when it came to gender), at times women and men's access to other types of capital was more important, for example, cultural capital. This perhaps reflects Rapps' (1998) argument that social class is important, but is much more complicated than is often portrayed.

Social class and screening

As Rapp (1998) points out, it is often assumed that working class women are more likely to reject prenatal testing whilst middle class women accept it uncritically. She shows that it is often not quite as straightforward. Certainly, within the context of this study many working class women accepted tests outright because they were offered. This can be seen in Rosie's account. Rosie was a housewife who had left school at 16. Her partner Pete was a self-employed plasterer who could not always find work. Despite their low economic and social capital, Rosie who was in the second trimester of pregnancy and her partner Pete accepted screening uncritically.

> We never questioned that we would participate, it's offered so you teke it. You might not always like the ways they do things but you have to go for it don't you.
>
> (Rosie, 27, Housewife)

Rosie's account was fairly common among other women who identified as working class. This can be seen again in Chelsea's account. Chelsea was in the third trimester of pregnancy. She was a care worker whose partner Rob worked in a factory. Both had left school at 16 with few formal qualifications. Again, Chelsea partook in all antenatal screening and did not think to question her participation:

> There was never any question that we would go for screening. It's just what you do isn't it?
>
> (Chelsea, 25, Care worker)

Several of the women in the study (who would be identified as traditionally 'working class' according to occupation and educational levels), accepted screening as part of their antenatal care package. This stands in opposition to some of the findings of existing studies which show that working class women are less likely to opt for prenatal care. Similarly, highly educated middle class women within this study did not always accept screening. Often women who rejected screening for Down's syndrome were highly educated middle class women. They tended to research the wider issues raised by screening in order to reach an informed decision. This can be seen in the account from Liz, a university researcher who held both undergraduate and postgraduate degrees:

> Well, we thought long and hard about the tests you know. Did lots of reading around the various issues and thought about what the implications of having a child with a disability might mean. We talked lot about it before we opted against *that* screening.
>
> (Liz, 32, University researcher)

This highlights some of the complexities of class that Rapp (1998) highlighted in her study on amniocentesis – that use of screening and testing could not be split straightforwardly according to whether you are middle or working class. It also highlights the importance of education and an individual's degree of cultural capital, thus reinforcing the importance of exploring the multifaceted aspects of social class. However, this is not to downplay the importance of socio-economic position. For example a couple's material resources also played a role in determining their access to certain types of screening. This was important when it came to opting for a nuchal fold scan. As already shown, nuchal fold (or translucency) scans were (at the time this study was conducted) not available free as part of local NHS antenatal care. Nuchal fold scans were available only privately at a cost of over one hundred pounds.[5] Due to this significant cost, the only couples to opt for this type of screening were those identifying as middle class, with high levels of economic and cultural capital. This can be seen in the account from Lucy, a hospital doctor, who opted for nuchal fold because of her knowledge and experience as a doctor and because she could afford it:

> We opted to have the Nuchal fold because we could. We knew more about it knew where we could get it. We are both doctors and knew the potential implications of having a baby once you've turned 35. I know it's not fair, I think it costs around £200 and lots of people wouldn't be able to afford it.
>
> (Lucy, 35, Hospital doctor)

Lucy's account emphasises the combined importance of economic, social and cultural capital in determining women's access to some types of tests. Lucy earned enough money to opt for the scan. She also held significant knowledge about the scan (what it was for, how it could increase risk prediction) through her work as doctor. Another respondent Eleanor who was degree educated, and a part-time director of a family business also opted for a nuchal fold scan. She also discussed the financial implications of this.

> With the nuchal fold, money was never an issue. We could afford it and I wanted to have it for reassurance so we did.
>
> (Eleanor, 34, Director of family company)

These accounts from middle class respondents can then be placed in contrast to the account from Emma who had left school at 16 and had worked as a nanny. Her partner was a soldier in the army. She did not know much about the benefits of nuchal fold and what it could do. She also could not afford it: 'Nuchal what? Yeah the midwife did say something I think, I can't remember. We wouldn't of paid for anything extra though as we don't have much money' (Emma, 22, Nanny).

These accounts from respondents on nuchal fold highlight the importance of material resources on women's ability to opt for extra screening such as nuchal fold. The economic aspects of class are therefore important in this context. However, they also illuminate the importance of cultural capital as respondents who were highly educated also tended to know more about nuchal fold screening than those who had left school at 16. This reinforces Rapp's (1998) argument that middle class women are often more comfortable than working class women with the scientific worldview on which the ethos of prenatal screening is based.

Social class, youth and antenatal clinic

Although there were no teenage parents in this study (the youngest respondent was aged 22), respondents in the study often made correlations between youth, social class and gender roles. This was based mostly on respondents' observations of young women in the antenatal clinic. Respondents in the study often discussed young single mums in the clinic identifying them as having little or no male involvement in prenatal care. This can be seen in the account from Sarah a school teacher who was in the second trimester of pregnancy:

> It's the young single mums I feel sorry for you know you see them in clinic. They look so young, some of them only look about 17 and they are already on their second child you know. I know it's a stereotype but they don't look as if they work. The clinic is packed with them. There's never a dad around, they are either alone or they bring their mums.
>
> (Sarah, 33, Teacher)

It was not just women respondents who made these observations but also men. This is also reflected in the account from Liz's partner Brendan:

> You see so many young single mums in clinic, with no dads, poor women. They don't seem to have anything, saddled with several kids no job no education. No partner to share things with.
>
> (Brendan, 33, Travel agent)

Sometimes respondents linked social class, with youth and access to antenatal classes. Antenatal classes are offered free as part of routine antenatal care on the NHS. These classes take place towards the later stages of pregnancy to help couples plan and prepare for labour and childbirth/care. Some of these classes and related parent-craft classes were aimed at all pregnant women and potential parents regardless of social background. Other classes, however, were run specifically for young couples, young fathers and single mums on low incomes. There were some respondents in this study who felt that the attendees of such groups were largely aged thirty plus and middle class. This was despite the intentions of the NHS to target those who were young and on low incomes. It was mostly the middle class, well-educated and informed couples who attended even though they perhaps did not really need to. This is articulated by Sean whose partner Kylie was in the second trimester of pregnancy:

> It is funny the antenatal classes were just full of all the wrong sort of people – all middle class sort of people and all the people who didn't need help because we had all read the books.
>
> (Sean, 30, Self-employed)

Again this was something that was identified by other respondents as can be seen in the account below from Sarah, a school teacher:

> We did try the NHS antenatal classes. I'm not being funny but we're both educated, and in our 30s and did lot of research on pregnancy, screening, childbirth, etc. ourselves. We didn't find out that much when we went except the tour of the labour ward was good. The people that probably really did it though, young mums and dads, those without much money, etc. they weren't there. I know they try to run extra groups extra for young dads to get them involved and that but you wonder whether anyone actually turns up.
>
> (Sarah, 33, Teacher)

Some respondents made correlations between class, gender and youth in antenatal clinic. These were mostly middle class respondents who were in their twenties or thirties themselves and who had supportive partners. Such respondents tended to identify young, poor single mothers as those who were least likely to access and make use of the appropriate antenatal care. Respondents also tended to feel that these young women were also least likely to have a supportive partner during pregnancy and childbirth. However, these observations were based on subjective accounts given by respondents interviewed; as this study did not include a focus on very young women, it is hard to comment more fully on this aspect of social class and screening.

Gender, work and screening

Through focusing on the impact of class on women and men's experiences of prenatal screening, the impact of class on gender roles was also explored. There appeared to be no differences in respondents' accounts according to social class and the level of emotional support men gave their partners. Men of all social classes attempted to attend prenatal screening appointments and wanted to be involved in their partners' pregnancy. This can be seen in the account from Chelsea, a care worker, and her partner Rob, a factory worker. Rob attended all hospital appointments and where possible tried to attend community appointments. Chelsea highlights the importance of his support:

> No I can't fault him, he does everything with me. He comes to all the appointments. He even takes annual leave so he can attend and he doesn't get much holiday. We're in this together and he wants to experience it all with me.
>
> (Chelsea, 25, Care worker)

Rob's desire for involvement in Chelsea's pregnancy and screening was no different to that articulated by respondents identifying as middle class. Lucy, a hospital doctor, aired similar views to Chelsea in discussing her own partner William's involvement: 'We make all decisions together and he's with me all the way. We're a team' (Lucy, 35, Hospital doctor).

The only area where class directly affected gender roles for respondents within this study was with regard to work constraints. This has already been explored to some extent in Chapter 2 on issues of choice and time. Men in semi or unskilled employment were often less likely to get time off from work to attend their partner's prenatal screening appointments. This was often more pronounced when men were in manual professions working on shifts. This often meant that the extent of their involvement varied according to their shift patterns. This can be seen in the account from Rebecca, a housewife who was married to Bill, an electrician: 'He does go to the hospital appointments, scans, with me. If he's on afternoons, then he will come. But obviously if he's working or anything he won't come' (Rebecca, 36, Housewife).

This account from Rebecca can again be placed in contrast with men from middle class professions whose ability to participate was greater given their increased access to flexible working patterns. This again was reflected in Lucy's account. Her partner William was a salaried GP who was able to get time off to attend her antenatal appointments: ' … It's difficult to get time off work and I'm quite fortunate that William is quite flexible, so generally he can come along to things … ' (Lucy, 35, Hospital doctor). This can also be seen in the account from Liz whose partner was a travel agent who worked flexible hours and was able to get time off.

> Yeah. I mean, it just seems very accepted that you go to these scans and you have time off work, I think we've been quite lucky with you getting time off work initially. Probably in some unlucky jobs it might be more difficult to. Yeah, I guess, I don't know what it would be like if you were a single person to be honest, that might be, if you were on your own. I wouldn't want to do it.
>
> (Liz, 32, University researcher)

Many respondents distinguished between types of antenatal appointments viewing some as more important than others. As argued in Chapter 3, those involving a 'picture of the baby', that is, ultrasound being the most important with routine community appointments being the least important. The ability for men to get time off work to accompany their partners to screening was often differentiated by occupational status. This can be seen in the account from Suzie, a wages clerk whose partner Ben worked in a fairly low-paid clerical job:

INTERVIEWER: Did he come with you to the hospital?

SUZIE: Yes, he came with me, yeah, he comes to the screening, and he came to those. But with the midwife, if it's only me being here for twenty minutes, seeing the midwife, doing a sort of routine. If something was wrong, if I felt that there was something not right, I would probably want him with me. But if it's just a routine appointment he's got to take time out of work, and it's not really that important that he's there.

(Suzie, 34, Housewife)

Social class did appear to play a role in respondents' attitudes towards an experience of screening. However, it is important that this role is not overestimated. Furthermore, in agreement with Rapp (1998), class influence here was not straightforwardly articulated in the ways often portrayed in existing literature, of working class women as screening refusers and middle class women as active accepters of screening. It was rather more complicated than that. Many working class women in this study happily participated in screening while some middle class women rejected it. This highlights not only the complexities of class influence but also that class influence involves a complex interweaving of cultural, social and economic capital. However, while the complexities of social class have been highlighted here the more traditional material aspects of class continue to play a role. For example, couples with limited economic capital were often unable to afford tests such as nuchal fold scans. The intersection of class, education and age was also reflected in the attitudes of some respondents toward young single mothers' engagements with antenatal care. Some female and male respondents held very strong, if somewhat stereotypical views on this issue. Finally, when it came to the impact of class on gender roles among respondents in this study class did not seem to have a significant influence. Both couples identifying as working and middle class were similar in their desire to take more equitable roles in screening. Where it did play a role, however, was in the context of work. As shown here (and in Chapter 2) men from manual and semi-skilled or unskilled occupations were often less able to participate in their partner's prenatal screening than those in skilled non-manual and professional employment. These men were less likely to have flexible working arrangements which facilitated their involvement. Therefore, in the context of gender perhaps age and economic capital have the biggest influence on roles. The issue of social class has been given extensive thought in this section; the second section of this chapter will move on to explore issues relating to race, ethnicity and screening.

Race, ethnicity and prenatal screening

The connections between race, ethnicity and certain genetic disorders have long been the centre of much discussion and debate. For example, inherited blood disorders are more common among people of African Caribbean and West African descent, Cypriots, South Asians and Chinese (Atkin, Ahmad and Anionwu 1998). A greater incidence of neural tube defects such as spina bifida have been reported among pregnant women of Mexican (and other Hispanic origin) descent (Browner *et al.* 1999). Furthermore, the metabolic disease Tay-Sachs (TSD) has been associated with Jewish populations of Ashkenazi descent (Wailoo and Pemberton 2006). These are all conditions that can be screened for prenatally (in the case of Tay-Sachs also pre-prenatally). In the UK, the connections between certain minority ethnic groups with inherited blood disorders have tended to lead to a focus in research on issues of discrimination in screening policy and practice. In particular, existing studies have highlighted the ethnic stereotyping and marginalisation of minority ethnic groups inherent in haemoglobinopathy screening services. Authors critiquing the selective nature of screening services highlight the potentially eugenicist nature of screening programmes (Dyson 1999). Research has also highlighted the ways in which screening professionals themselves may not always be adequately trained to deal with the connections between inherited blood disorders and certain minority ethnic groups (Dyson 1995). Several studies further highlight the low priority of haemoglobinopathy screening and services, linking this to broader issues of racist service provision (Atkin, Ahmad and Anionwu 1998).

When it comes to screening for Down's syndrome and other chromosomal or structural anomalies research has tended to focus on issues of access to screening and diagnostic testing. Rowe *et al.* (2008) for example as shown earlier found that ethnicity and social class significantly affected the likelihood of patients being offered ultrasound and amniocentesis screening for

Down's syndrome. According to existing research, Black and minority ethnic women are also less likely to opt for screening and testing for Down's syndrome. On exploring the attitudes of pregnant Saudi Arabian women towards screening for Down's syndrome Babay (2004) found a higher acceptance of non-invasive methods. Of those participants who accepted the idea of screening (61.1%) 'all accepted ultrasound screening', whilst acceptance of the invasive procedures was far lower (34.2%) (p. 5). These findings have been confirmed by studies on various ethnic minority communities in the US, for example, Mexican origin and black women are less likely than white and other populations to use amniocentesis (Brett *et al.* 1994, Browner *et al.* 1999).

Cultural differences in women's attitudes towards pregnancy are one of the most frequently cited reasons used to explain women's low take-up of all screening services. For example, Barnes and Boddy (1994) argue that within Somali culture lay perceptions of pregnancy and childbirth are viewed as a natural and spiritual event, not a medical one therefore Somali women tend to eschew these types of technologies. Kuppermann *et al.* (1996) further suggest that cultural variation in attitudes towards disability may also account for some ethnic differences in the use of screening technology. Religion is often cited as a key factor in ethnic minority women's refusal of prenatal technology. For example, women whose fetus may have been identified through routine screening as having problems often do not go to the extra tests they are referred to because they believe everything is in the hands of God. This is tied up with the anti-abortion views of certain religions (Lewando-Hundt *et al.* 2001: 576). Similarly certain understandings of the Koran may suggest that abortion is possible within the first 120 days of pregnancy if the mother's health is endangered (Panter-Brick 1991).

Racial discrimination and socio-economic factors are also crucially important. Racial harassment and discrimination are known factors in explaining health disparities between ethnic groups (Nazroo 2003). In the context of prenatal screening discriminatory practices cited in studies are wide ranging. For example traditional clothing such as the *hijab* or the *nikab* were found to lead to ethnic stereotyping by health professionals in Tsianakas and Liamputtong's (2002) study on Muslim women and maternity care in Australia. Women also often experience discrimination based on issues of language and poor communication (Bowler 1993; Reitmanova and Gustafson 2008). As argued earlier other authors such as Rapp (1994) have pointed to the class-based nature of racial discrimination in the prenatal arena. She argues that genetic counselling around prenatal screening is more in keeping with a white middle class world view, thus ethnic minority women from lower socioeconomic backgrounds are less likely to access and use these services.

The aim of this section of the chapter is to explore the impact of race and ethnicity on women and men's experiences of prenatal screening. The first part of this section will explore respondents' experiences and views on issues of race and racism in the prenatal clinic. The chapter will move on to explore ethnicity and attitudes to screening, impact of ethnicity and race on gender roles and the role of whiteness in screening. Overall, differences in this study according to race and ethnicity did not appear to be as significant as perhaps thought. The biggest issue raised in the context of respondents' accounts related to the issue of 'whiteness' and the distancing of ethnically white respondents from blood screening for inherited blood disorders. This racial distancing by respondents perhaps further reinforces the racialisation of health argument as applied to certain types of illness and disease (Reed 2003, 2011b). Before going on to explore the data two issues must be noted. First, the complexities of the use of concepts such as 'race' and ethnicity', while hierarchical, immutable categories of 'race' are no longer explicitly used to differentiate between groups, many features of racial thinking have permeated concepts of ethnicity and culture and negative connotations have been applied to certain ethnic or cultural groups of people (Ahmad and Bradby 2007). This chapter acknowledges the need to move away from negative associations based on 'ethnic groups' drawing instead on a dynamic and culturally situated notion of ethnicity (Reed 2003). Second, it is important to note methodological limitations in this context as only a small number of respondents within the study identified as Black and minority ethnic. Therefore explorations and arguments relating to these issues are tentative.

Race and racism in the clinic

Black, South Asian and Mauritian respondents in the study and some of the white respondents did talk to some extent about issues of race, ethnicity and racism in the antenatal clinic. Black and minority ethnic respondents did not discuss the issue of racism overtly. This could of course relate to the race of interviewer effect. Both interviewers were ethnically white and this could have impacted on whether minority ethnic respondents felt comfortable speaking about issues of race to a white interviewer (Rhodes 1994). Nonetheless, respondents here tended to mention it opaquely as can be seen in the account from a Black African respondent Jameela who was in the third trimester of pregnancy:

> Well, I wouldn't say that the midwives were racist. I felt like they certainly weren't surprised when I tested positive for sickle cell. It's almost like with me being a black African they expect it. On the whole though I've got no complaints about my treatment.
>
> (Jameela, 37, Student accountant)

This view was similarly shared in accounts given by Pinky, a south Asian respondent, who was in the second trimester of pregnancy and had tested positive for the thalassaemia trait:

> I was treated really well during screening, especially when my blood tests showed up positive (for thalassaemia). The midwives couldn't have been

> nicer to me or my husband but then we are both British born ... when I look at some of the Muslim women in clinic, the Somalis that don't speak English, I wonder just how well they get treated?
>
> (Pinky, 30, Bank clerk)

Again Pinky's account reinforces some of the arguments made by Puthussery *et al.* (2008) in their work on the differences in attitudes of health professionals towards British-born Asian women and those who are first generation. The issue at the centre of this is language and whether English is an individual's first or second language. Numerous studies have focused on the impact of language in the antenatal setting (Bowler 1993). In the context of this study, there was only one respondent, Katarina, who was Czech who raised language as a problem.

> The midwives were brilliant when I went for my tests. They did keep asking me to repeat things, because I am Czech English is not my first language. This was a bit annoying because I think I speak English pretty well!
>
> (Katarina, 28, Self-employed)

Some respondents raised issues of racial discrimination and stereotyping and language barriers similar to those highlighted in other studies. However, as argued earlier samples were so small it is hard to comment in detail on this issue. Furthermore, the sample was perhaps biased as all respondents selected were active users of antenatal health services who accepted prenatal screening. It would be interesting to explore accounts of women from minority ethnic groups in more detail who had rejected screening. However, those involved in further screening such as Jameela and Pinky did not seem to feel that they were direct recipients of racism in the clinic.

Along with respondents identifying as black and minority ethnic, some white respondents commented on issues of race and racism in the clinic. Some white respondents observed racist incidents in the antenatal clinic and discussed these during their interviews. For example, Sarah, a white respondent in the third trimester of pregnancy, in particular felt very ashamed at the treatment of a Black British woman by a midwife while Sarah herself was in the clinic for a screening appointment.

> Well, I was outraged. There was this black woman in clinic. Actually I think she had come in for diabetes testing. Anyway, the midwife calls her name and comes up to her, speaks really slowly as if she's stupid and says, 'do you speak English'. I felt like bloody shouting, of course she bloody speaks English, she is British. She has obviously lived here all our life. Honestly, I was so embarrassed I didn't know whether to ignore it or whether to say something. My partner was a bit worried I was going to march over a give 'em a piece of my mind.
>
> (Sarah, 33, Teacher)

A number of studies have highlighted this issue of ethnic stereotyping in the prenatal clinic. Studies have tended to show that midwives working in antenatal clinic tend to make unconscious assumptions based on racial/ethnic stereotyping (Atkin, Ahmad and Anionwu 1998; Rowe and Garcia 2005), an example of which is that Muslim women do not want prenatal diagnosis (Modell *et al.* 2000; Rowe and Garcia 2005). Puthussery *et al.* (2008) argue that often midwives make assumptions based on whether ethnic minority women are British born or not. They are also more likely to treat British-born ethnic minority women in similar ways to white women. This perhaps can be seen in Sarah's observations in the prenatal arena.

Ethnicity and attitudes to serum screening

Existing literature on ethnicity and screening for Down's syndrome has tended to explore differences across groups in attitudes towards disability. Learman *et al.* (2003) show that although Down's syndrome screening does not involve the potential for racial/ethnic stigmatisation that can occur in the context of screening/testing for conditions such as Tay-Sachs disease or inherited blood disorders, the experiences of some groups may have important impacts on current attitudes towards testing (Moyer *et al.* 1999). Some studies show that the type of information given and the way women were informed about the test had more impact on women's decision-making than did either their ethnic or social background (Press and Browner 1994). Other studies have identified modest variation across ethnic groups on women's attitudes towards testing and decision-making (Learman *et al.* 2003). Again, although sample size was small, Black, South Asian and Mauritian women in this study tended to accept screening for Down's syndrome in the same ways that most white respondents did. This can be seen in the account from Pinky:

PINKY: We had all the tests both sets yes. Erm I didn't think too much about the differences really I just wanted a healthy baby so anything that could check for that was all I cared about. Obviously because I tested positive for thalassaemia that became a bit of a sticking point.

INTERVIEWER: What do you mean?

PINKY: Well, once that happened I was more concerned about that than the other routine tests.

INTERVIEWER: So were you not as concerned about screening for Down's syndrome.

PINKY: Not at that point no.

(Pinky, 30, Bank clerk)

As argued earlier, although Black, South Asian and Mauritian respondents tended to have more experience with testing for inherited blood disorders as shown in other studies too (Rapp 2000), women also wanted to be involved in screening for other issues such as Down's. This is reflected in the account below from Jameela:

> No I didn't feel differently about the tests. I had them all. Obviously I had more personal experience with sickle cell but I approached all the tests in the same way, I had every test they offered including the one for Down's syndrome.
>
> (Jameela, 37, Student accountant)

As shown throughout the book, there was one British Mauritian respondent Flo who had received a risky test result for Down's syndrome for both her pregnancies and went on subsequently to have an amniocentesis. Although in both cases the amniocentesis showed that the baby did not have Down's syndrome. Flo did not feel her cultural background influenced her decision, rather her own experience of working with people with disabilities played a major role in her decision-making process:

> Oh, there was never any question that I would have all the blood tests no. We just took it for granted that we would go through all the screening. When it came to the amniocentesis that was a bit more difficult, weighing up whether we could cope with a child who had disabilities. Knowing what we know, with the job we do, it's hard.
>
> (Flo, 35, Self-employed)

Issues of ethnicity did not seem to factor particularly strongly in Black, South Asian and Mauritian respondents' decisions about screening for Down's syndrome screening. This perhaps supports the findings of some existing studies that have highlighted the importance of other factors (e.g. partners) over ethnicity in influencing decision-making (Press and Browner 1993). This was, however, not necessarily the case for ethnically white respondents as will be explored in the following section.

Haemoglobinopathy screening and 'whiteness'

As argued throughout this book inherited blood disorders are more likely to occur in particular populations. Statistics show significant variation in positive carrier rates between ethnic groups with 1.85 per 1000 in those babies recorded as white British compared to 145 per 1000 African babies (Streetly *et al.* 2010). Due to the low risk of white British populations being identified as carriers of the sickle or thalassaemia trait, research has tended not to focus on the impact of inherited blood disorders on white British women and men. However, white people can be and are carriers of sickle and thalassaemia trait (there was one white respondent in this study who was a thalassaemia carrier). However, most white respondents within this study tended to assume that their ethnicity placed them as low risk of being carriers and therefore distanced themselves from this screening. This can be seen in the account below from Joanne, who was in the second trimester of pregnancy:

> We were asked for consent about whether we wanted to have all these things and I am quite.I think I am quite well informed about quite a lot of things anyway about biology and screening. … I didn't really feel like I needed to ask questions but I think my partner did. Things like the thalassaemia I know that we have a very very slim chance of having that because it tends not to be found in white people.
>
> (Joanne, 35, Nurse)

Other respondents used their whiteness to reinforce this 'racial' distancing from screening for inherited blood disorders. They often did not worry as much about screening for blood disorders as they felt that because they were white, it would not affect them. Again as articulated by Zoe:

> It's just because it was offered and it was only blood, and I think as well that they (tests for inherited blood disorders) are only sort of cut and dry. It was like you have the blood test and they would say 'yes you've got it' or 'no you haven't', and they were sort of, quite, not minor conditions, but not necessarily major disabilities. And also they were quite unlikely, like the sickle cell thing, it was unlikely for a white person to have it, it's not common. Yeah, it was just they were just taking blood for a lot of other reasons, it just didn't seem like a problem.
>
> (Zoe, 31, Museums officer)

This racial distancing from screening for blood disorders by ethnically white respondents was then placed in contrast to their fears over screening for Down's syndrome which respondents often felt could happen to anyone regardless of ethnicity. This can be seen in the account from Christine who was in the third trimester of pregnancy below:

> Yes, I suppose maybe the sickle cell and thalassaemia seem more routine and they don't happen to many white people. Maybe the Down's has more impact and you have to sort of make your decision based on that. But yeah, looking back, that was when I was more concerned about it.
>
> (Christine, 34, IT consultant)

There was only one ethnically white respondent Emma who appeared concerned about her chances of carrying the sickle or thalassaemia trait, and in articulating her concerns over it also discussed the implications for her partner. Most white respondents did not speak in such detail on these issues:

> I said to him I'm having all these tests done. Obviously when you have your thalassaemia test, if mine comes back positive it doesn't mean that the baby's going to have it but I have to find out if my partner's a carrier too, so he has to be tested. So obviously we talked about that, so then we discussed everything, like we discussed whether we wanted to know the

sex and did we want to know if it had Down's syndrome and you know stuff like that, and he agreed, so yeah we had a conversation about it.

(Emma, 22, Nanny)

There was one respondent, Sarah who tested border-line positive for thalassaemia who was very shocked that she tested positive for this trait because she felt that her 'whiteness' gave her some kind of protection from it.

INTERVIEWER: Were you surprised then to get a positive result for the thalassaemia test?

SARAH: Er yes I was actually because we were led to believe it didn't really apply to us, being white.

(Sarah, 33, Teacher)

While Black, South Asian and Mauritian respondents did not appear to distinguish significantly between types of screening and accepted all screening, white respondents tended to racially distance themselves from blood screening for inherited blood disorders. There is of course a materiality to this issue as statistically white people are much less likely to either carry the trait or gene or develop these disorders (Streetly *et al.* 2010). However, it can and does happen. Therefore two other issues can be observed in this context: first, the accounts from the study highlight the importance of recognising whiteness as a practised racialised identity which informs respondents' views on screening. Second, the accounts from the white respondents in this study emphasised the continued racial associations of blood disorders with certain populations leading to the continuance of a racialisation of health.

Race, ethnicity and gender roles in screening

Rapp (1998) found in her study on amniocentesis that men's influence over women and their involvement in screening directly reflected men's own racial and cultural experiences. For example she uses one case from her study where an African American male did not want his pregnant partner to participate in the amniocentesis test. His position was not merely an exertion of male domination and female subordination but as Rapp (1998) argues was a reflection of his views on the history of race, science and medicine. When given the consent form for testing which talks about using biological material drawn for research he refers back to broader historical experiences of African Americans being used for scientific experiments. A good example of this was shown in the famous 1970s US Public Health study of untreated syphilis in Macon County (known as the Tuskegee syphilis experiment) where the deterioration of black men's health through failure to treat was observed by researchers all in the name of scientific progress (Wailoo 2001). Historical examples of racial experimentation such as these informed this particular respondent's beliefs on his partner's involvement in amniocentesis. Rapp (1998) is clear to highlight in her study that gender roles in this context are not straightforward. It was not a simple case of male domination and women's subordination, or male insistence on female difference, but the disruption of not quite conscious gender assumptions that relatively new technology such as amniocentesis brings to the surface.

It is impossible to generalise on issues of ethnicity and gender in this context due to the limitations of the study. Certainly, what was highlighted earlier in Chapter 5 was the ways in which black and minority ethnic respondents who were involved in positive screening for blood disorders espoused equitable gender roles as men were also involved in screening. However, what happened when it came to routine screening? When it came to routine screening and antenatal appointments Black and Asian respondents continued to articulate equal gender roles. This can be seen in the account below from Jameela:

> Obviously he came with me for the sickle cell testing and he came to clinic on a separate occasion to be tested himself. When it came to screening for Down's syndrome I went alone because it was at the GPs not the hospital and he couldn't get time off. He was very supportive though and we made decisions about the tests together.
>
> (Jameela, 37, Student accountant)

As argued earlier, Jameela's partner Tunde who also identified as Black African was very supportive during her positive screening for sickle cell anaemia and was subsequently screened himself. However, he was also supportive during routine screening and antenatal care more generally. This can be seen in the quote below:

> I tried to go to as many of her appointments as I could. I wanted to be supportive. She has to do all the hard work (laughs!) but I don't want to feel she's alone.
>
> (Tunde, 37, Pyschiatrist)

The importance of male participation was also highlighted by Pinky's partner Bihar who was also South Asian. He not only discussed his support during her positive screening result for thalassaemia but also discussed his involvement in her pregnancy more generally.

> Do you know that I really enjoyed her pregnancy and I wanted to be involved. It was really scary when she tested positive for thalassaemia but you know we took it in our stride together. We talked about all the tests together as a couple not just the blood testing, although to be honest that stayed in our minds for a long time.
>
> (Bihar, 31, Shop owner)

One final issue to explore before concluding this chapter is the role of whiteness on gender roles. There were specific examples within the study where whiteness played a particular role in informing gender roles. This was again in relation to blood screening for inherited blood disorders. White male respondents often knew less about screening for blood disorders and also distanced themselves from the possibility of being carriers of the sickle cell or thalassaemia trait due to their ethnic whiteness. They were often therefore less likely to engage with this aspect of their partners' screening. This is highlighted in the account from Bill, whose partner Rebecca was in the second trimester of pregnancy:

BILL: Well, I know she had some tests done. I went with her and everything. I know one of them was for HIV and I think that some were for blood problems. I knew more about the Down's one though at 15 weeks. We were both worried about that but to be honest we weren't worried about those earlier ones.
INTERVIEWER: Why was that?
BILL: Well, they don't happen to people like us do they?
INTERVIEWER: Can I ask what you mean by that?
BILL: Well, white people. Whereas Down's, that can happen to anyone

(Bill, 37, Electrician)

In one specific case this racial distancing through whiteness led one male respondent to opt not to be screened for thalassaemia. Paul was Flo's partner. He was the only male respondent in the study not to be screened despite his partner's positive result. In his interview he reinforces the issue of whiteness as a reason not to be screened. As Paul's quote shows:

PAUL: Well we didn't see much point in me being tested as the potential for me having it was low. I would have been happy to but Flo felt there was no need.
INTERVIEWER: Do you mind me asking why that was?
PAUL: Well, I don't know much about but isn't it that white people don't really get it?

(Paul, 31, Self-employed)

This then gives one example whereby whiteness has a direct impact on gender and in particular on men's roles. As argued earlier, however, it was too difficult in this study to tease out in particular the impact of ethnicity on issues of gender due to the skewed nature of the sample. Gender roles across all ethnic groups involved in the study mostly reinforced similar patterns which emphasised the shift towards men's increased roles in pregnancy and screening on the one hand, whilst continuing to reflect traditional gender roles on the other. Further work is required on this issue particularly around perhaps haemoglobinopathy screening and whiteness. With the rise in relationships between men and women across different ethnic groups, white male participation in screening may become increasingly important.

Conclusion

There has been much debate in existing literature over whether new genetic technologies challenge or reinforce existing forms of inequality. While some have emphasised the role of individual choice in enabling these technologies to transform existing social relations, others have suggested that these technologies both reinforce and actually create new forms of inequality. This chapter has focused on exploring whether these technologies transform existing inequalities or reinforce them focusing in particular on issues of social class and race and ethnicity. The chapter has also explored the ways in which gender roles in screening may be mediated by both social class and race and ethnicity. Drawing on the accounts from respondents in this study, the same arguments can be made as having been articulated with regard to gender. The prenatal screening arena does present a forum from which to challenge existing inequalities of social class and race and ethnicity. However, it also to an extent reinforces them; the outcome therefore is somewhat of a paradox.

The first half of the chapter showed that while there were some differences in respondents' attitudes towards screening across social class, these were far less pronounced than is often presented in existing literature in the field. Social class differences were quite subtle and often involved a complex interweaving of women's access to and use of different types of capital – economic, social, cultural and symbolic. For example, while women across all social classes took part in screening, for women who identified as working class this involvement was automatic. However, often middle class women were more likely to interrogate the process, using their cultural capital to inform their approach to decision-making (Rapp 1998). While respondents' accounts tended to highlight the importance of taking a multifaceted approach to social class, the importance of the material aspects of class were never far from the surface. For example women's ability to opt for private tests such as nuchal fold scans was often curtailed by economic constraints. When it came to gender roles social class appeared to have a limited impact. It seemed mostly that men across social classes all wanted to be involved in their partner's prenatal care. Where social class did have an impact on gender roles this was mostly related again to economic and occupational aspects of class. Men in semi or unskilled occupations wanted to be as involved as men in skilled and professional occupations but often could not afford to take time off to attend or lacked work flexibility to be able to do so. Therefore, while class differences existed, they were not the only or indeed most important factor in determining women and men's experiences of prenatal screening.

The second half of the chapter focused on exploring issues relating to race, ethnicity and screening. As argued earlier, there has been a significant amount of research and writing on the issue of race, ethnicity and screening and ethnicity and antenatal care in general both in the UK and US. Most existing literature has argued that women from minority ethnic backgrounds are less likely to be offered screening than white women and are also less likely to use antenatal services. This has mostly been related by existing research to ethnic stereotyping and other issues of racial discrimination in the health services. Existing studies have also highlighted differences in attitudes towards screening across ethnic groups, emphasising cultural differences in attitudes towards issues of disability. Drawing on respondents' accounts in this study discrimination did not seem to play a massive role in women's experiences of screening. As already argued throughout this book, Black, South Asian and Mauritian respondents were particularly knowledgeable about screening for blood disorders in comparison to white respondents. However, when it came to serum screening for chromosomal anomalies, no real differences were observed across differing ethnic groups. Black, South Asian and Mauritian respondents within the study tended to exhibit equal gender roles in their experiences of both problematic and routine screening. However, throughout the study many ethnically white men were also involved in their partner's screening. Where there were differences between men this related to many other issues such as work, family, etc. not to issues of ethnicity explicitly (Press and Browner 1993).

One issue of particular interest here related to the role of 'whiteness' as an ethnic identity and screening for inherited blood disorders. Ethnically white respondents tended to 'racially' distance themselves from this type of screening during interviews. This appeared to emphasise two issues: first, the accounts from the study highlighted the importance of recognising whiteness as a practised racialised identity which informs respondents' views on screening. Second, the accounts from the white respondents in this study emphasised the continued racial associations of blood disorders with certain populations leading to the continuance of a racialisation of health around blood disorders. As shown by some studies, assumptions made by professionals about white people not being at risk of carrying the thalassaemia trait has led in some cases to couples not being offered screening and unknowingly going on to have a baby with thalassaemia (Atkin, Ahmad and Anionwu 1998). The need therefore for further research on this particular issue is perhaps required.

Overall, the respondents' accounts in this study present the screening arena as a place where social inequality is both challenged and reinforced. To what extent inequalities according to class and race however relates to the use of the technology in its own right and how much they merely reflect existing social divisions is unknown. The idea that prenatal screening itself can transform social divisions rests on an assumption that it is a neutral piece of technology, an equaliser open to individual choice. However as Mitchell and Georges (1997) have shown in their study on fetal ultrasound in Greece and Canada, while fetal ultrasound is often presented in popular and professional discourses across the globe as a passive and neutral technology, the image of the fetus shown using such technology is actually imbued with cultural meanings by both potential parents and professionals. Prenatal technologies therefore are already themselves social and culturally inscribed not blank scripts.

Furthermore, according to Webster (2007: 89) for new medical technologies such as prenatal screening to have any significant effect on economic inequality, they would need to bring about one or more of the following: a redistribution of socio-economic (including health) resources in a more equitable way; the provision of new resources to empower previously disadvantaged groups improving their overall life chances; or challenge the existing socio-economic distribution of resources. For Webster (2007: 89) these changes would need to be implemented in such a way so that the outcome had systematic rather than random effects. This is unlikely to occur in this existing financial climate. Overall, most new health technologies have a limited impact on patterns of inequality, even when they can be shown to have positive clinical outcomes at the level of the patient (Webster 2007). Health problems linked to individual social inequality may not be seen to result from their engagements with new technologies such as prenatal screening. Rather they are experienced in a more direct sense; by simply the feeling of being unwell or ill (Webster 2007: 91). This argument does perhaps explain the limited impact of new technologies more broadly on patterns of social inequality. However, the picture painted in context of this chapter and small-scale study is hopefully not quite so bleak. Although the transformative potential of the technology itself is perhaps limited, as shown within the context of prenatal screening, social inequalities can be both challenged and reinforced. This is through the use of such technology by women and men within and across varying social positions. Having explored broader issues of stratification and screening within this chapter, the following final chapter of the book will return to the main focus of the book on gender roles. In doing so it aims to offer an overall evaluation of the book's initial aims, further exploring future possibilities in the screening arena.

Conclusion

Introduction

The focus of this book has been on exploring gender roles in prenatal blood screening. In particular the aim has been to explore both women and men's roles during screening for inherited blood disorders and screening for chromosomal anomalies. As shown in the introduction, little attention has been given in existing research to men's roles in screening – both as supportive partners of women undergoing screening and as direct recipients of screening themselves. Drawing on data from a qualitative study on gender roles and responsibilities in screening, this book has aimed to address this gap in existing research, providing an exploration of the gendered nature of genetic screening. This final chapter has two key aims: first, through close examination of the findings of the study the conclusion will focus an evaluation of gender roles during the process of screening. It will return here to some of the original questions asked at the start of the book such as: to what extent men are involved in screening, how advantageous is this for both men and women? The findings of the study will be evaluated in the context of broader patterns of gender-related social change. Second, the conclusion will assess whether men can/should be more involved in this process, and if so how. The chapter will pay particular attention here to the various institutional, organisational and ideological changes required for further male involvement. The chapter will also include reflections on the original theoretical framework of gender role ideology outlined at the start of the book.

The conclusion will begin with an examination of gender roles in screening as highlighted in the findings of the study. As noted throughout the book, screening does seem to emphasise traditional views on pregnancy. However, it is also representative of significant changes in gender roles as men become more active participants in pregnancy and screening – including taking responsibility for their own genetic input into the health of the fetus. The chapter will move on to situate the findings of the study within the broader context of gender-related social change. As will be argued, gender roles highlighted here are indicative of gender roles in contemporary British society more generally – as existing gender roles continue to be publicly and privately both reinforced and challenged (Reed 2006). The latter sections of the chapter will move on to explore whether men can and should be more involved in screening. This will include a further evaluation of respondents' views along with an exploration of screening policy, practice and ideology.

Prenatal screening and the paradox of gender

This book started off with a number of questions to be addressed. In particular the aim was to explore the nature of gender roles in prenatal screening with a focus on both women and men. Did they reflect a traditional set of gender roles? To what extent did they signify significant changes? Were men's roles in screening evidence of a transition to the 'new father'? Did men and women share roles and responsibilities in screening? What does this mean for women's reproductive autonomy? Rapp (2000) has argued that prenatal screening and diagnosis acts as a forum for the making and re-making of gender roles. According to her, screening marks a resilient start for a set of parenting roles based on a traditional gender division of labour. However, the findings from this study highlighted a complex picture. While screening does seem to emphasise traditional views on pregnancy, it is also representative of significant changes in gender roles as men become more active participants in pregnancy and screening. Furthermore, the connection between gender and genetics itself is complex and contradictory as men both reinforce patriarchal ideologies around paternal genetics connections, whilst also taking more genetic 'paternal' responsibility. Throughout the book therefore a paradoxical set of gender roles has been highlighted.

Lorber (1994) argues that gender is paradoxical because, as she states when examined closely, much of what we take for granted about gender and its causes and effects either does not hold up or can be explained differently. One of the paradoxes of gender for her relates directly to gender and reproduction. It is often assumed that genetic or physiological differences between women and men lead to gender inequalities. However, she argues that females have the greater advantage over men in reproduction as they have the ability to give birth, thus according to her it is the institutions of gender that structure the unequal relations of reproduction not the other way around. This book has emphasised a set of gender paradoxes in prenatal screening. It highlights the push towards greater parity of gender roles in screening, whilst also emphasising ideological and institutional barriers which continue to circumscribe traditional views on gender, pregnancy and genetics. It also emphasises the need to encourage male participation whilst not losing site of women's reproductive autonomy, or the material constraints of pregnancy itself. This set of paradoxes is highlighted throughout various chapters of the book.

In Chapter 1 for example, the complexities of gender are clearly demonstrated through an exploration of information seeking and disseminating. The chapter highlights the ways in which women sought out information about pregnancy and genetic screening and selectively disseminated it to their male partners, thus reinforcing their role as guardians of the fetus. This was a role as shown in the chapter that was further reinforced by midwives and other health professionals who tended to disseminate screening information predominantly to women. However, the chapter also highlighted the ways in which this female exclusivity was currently being challenged by an increase in men's access to information about genetic screening (Locock and Alexander 2006), particularly through men's use of the Internet. Men used the Internet to seek out information on pregnancy, screening and genetic conditions. This allows them access to a previously exclusive female world, thus challenging women's roles as exclusive guardians of fetal health. The gender roles highlighted here therefore were paradoxical, emphasising both the push away from traditional gender roles in reproduction whilst also reinforcing them.

Chapter 2 also highlighted the complex nature of gender roles in screening with a specific focus on the issues of choice and time. Drawing on data from the study, the chapter emphasised the intersections between gender, choice and time in prenatal screening. As discussed, throughout screening women and men make choices, choices are gendered, routinised and placed in a set of temporal constraints. Women are constrained by their own corporeality as screening for genetic conditions and chromosomal anomalies must take place during certain periods of gestation. Men are constrained by social and institutional barriers – such as workplace norms that discourage them from taking time off to participate in screening (Williams and Umberson 1999). The very notion of reproductive 'choice' in this study therefore appears to be mediated and constrained by gender, time and materiality.

Gender roles within the study tended to vary according to the screening type used. As shown in Chapter 3 for example, both women and men distinguished between blood screening and ultrasound scans. Both saw the scans as more important in detecting genetic conditions and fetal anomalies because they gave visual evidence of the health of the fetus. This supports the findings of other studies which highlight the importance of the visual in Western culture, and which often locate lay understandings of genes (inheritance) with visual markers such as physical resemblance (Keller and Grontkowski 1983; Hall *et al.* 2007). In the context of this study, a particular set of gender roles tended to be mapped onto distinctions in screening type. Women and their DNA were associated with serum screening, men and their genes were associated with ultrasound. This chapter reaffirms the existence of the gendered nature of genetics and reproduction outlined at the start of the introduction to this book. Men's physical role in pregnancy may be primarily related to their presence at conception, as they subsequently become divorced from the day-to-day material realities of pregnancy itself. However, visual technologies enable them to reconnect biologically with their offspring (Sandelowski 1994). Furthermore, while men are reconnected physically to the fetus, these differences in technology serve to reinforce women's secondary role in genetic progress as fetal containers (Ettorre 2000).

The issue of gender and screening decision-making was explored in Chapter 4. This chapter showed that while men are now more involved in decision-making, in most cases men do not exert male control over women. For most couples in the study women continued to have the ultimate say in decision-making. As was argued in the chapter, this is something that continues to be reinforced by health professionals in the screening environment. It would appear therefore that women's reproductive autonomy is sustained despite men's participation in decision-making. Furthermore, while men's responsibility is increased in screening, especially when they are screened themselves, their roles continue to be viewed for the most part as secondary to those of the mother. This could perhaps be viewed as evidence of the feminist ideal in screening, reflecting the achievement of greater male responsibility without the loss of women's reproductive rights (Markens, Browner and Preloran 2003). However, men's secondary role could also be seen in this context as an example of the discrepancy between the culture and conduct of fatherhood as discussed earlier. Wall and Arnold (2007) for example highlight the ways in which the idea of 'the new fatherhood' is in fact an 'ideal' not yet fully realised in practice. While cultural understandings of both fatherhood and masculinity are multiple, fluid and changing (Lupton and Barclay 1997), the idea of fathers who are as equally involved with childrearing as mothers continues to clash with the hegemonic cultural ideals of masculinity (Connell 2000). This is perhaps reflected in respondents' accounts over issues of decision-making.

Chapter 5 explored the paradoxes of gender with a more direct focus on genetics. This chapter highlighted the gendered association of so-called 'good' and 'bad' genes in prenatal screening. As the findings of the study showed, men were often concerned with the establishment of 'good' genetic connections between themselves and the fetus. This reinforces the patriarchal view of paternity as outlined in the introduction to the book, of men as 'seed' as 'life' givers (Rothman 1986). Women in contrast often take responsibility for 'risky' screening results thus reinforcing their roles as nurturers (Ettorre 2002). However, the chapter again highlighted the complexities of gender roles and genetics. Maternal responsibility for the production of 'bad' genes is not straightforward but is complexly mediated by a number of other factors including ethnicity and screening type (Reed 2009a). Furthermore, at times men did take responsibility for the production of faulty genes in screening, particularly when they were direct participants in screening. Thus when it came to the gendering of good and bad genes, gender roles were paradoxical, simultaneously challenging and reinforcing a traditional gender division of labour.

The final two substantive chapters of the book situated the exploration of gender roles in a broader social context. Chapter 6 moved beyond an immediate focus on couples' experiences to explore the roles of family and friends. As shown through the findings of the study, friends often influenced couples' decisions to opt for certain types of prenatal screening. Family also affected screening decisions and occasionally led to disagreement between women and men. However, family influence in screening also has a more direct influence on genetics and gender roles (Rapp 2000). As shown within the chapter, respondents often had a general awareness that family genetic history can inform health outcomes. At times this awareness of history affected attitudes towards prenatal screening – particularly in cases where family members suffered from various inherited disorders. Family history also had direct clinical implications when genetic links were identified, sought out and monitored. Overall, the chapter emphasised the mostly positive roles played by family and friends in couples' experiences of prenatal screening – both indirectly through supporting women and their partners during screening and more directly through family history and inheritance. However, it also emphasised the primary significance of male partners' roles in this context. Furthermore, as data showed women often took the major responsibility for family genetic history thus reinforcing the gendered nature of genetics.

The final substantive chapter moved away from focusing explicitly on gender roles in screening in order to examine broader issues of class, race and ethnicity. This chapter focused on exploring the transformative potential of prenatal screening. Drawing on data from the study, along with a wider body of literature on inequality and screening, this chapter argued that technologies such as prenatal screening do present some challenges to existing forms of inequality. As shown through the data, while some social divisions existed between respondents these differences were perhaps not as pronounced as those highlighted in existing research. Furthermore, new issues relating to ethnicity were raised in the context of this study. These perhaps require further analysis in future research, for example, the role 'whiteness' plays as a racial distancing mechanism in the context of prenatal screening for inherited blood disorders. Overall, women and men's roles in prenatal screening in this study both challenged and reflected existing forms of stratification – including class, ethnicity and race. The chapter concluded by cautioning against the ability of genetic technology such as prenatal screening in itself being able to transform social relationships.

In answer to initial questions set out in the introduction, the book has shown that gender roles in screening and in reproduction are often complex, contradictory and in transition. While women continue to bear the brunt of responsibility for pregnancy and screening this is not exclusively the case as men take on more roles during this process as partners and potential fathers. Where men were involved directly in screening, they also shared some of the material burdens of pregnancy with women. This has the potential to shift the gendered associations of women and pregnancy, posing a further challenge to the existing gendered nature of reproductive genetics. However, while men's roles have increased, both women and men's roles continue to be mediated by broader social circumstances, by family friends, class, race and ethnicity. Furthermore, accounts from respondents continue to lend support to earlier arguments made over the influence of the institutions of gender which continue to place constraints on gender-related social change. The kinds of gender roles emphasised by the findings of this study in the context of prenatal screening must not be viewed in isolation. As will be shown in the following section, they are directly reflective of broader trends in gender relations.

Gender roles in screening, a snapshot of a broader context

The complexity of men's roles highlighted in the prenatal arena is indicative of the diverse and fluid nature of masculinity articulated within contemporary Western society (Robinson 2008). Relations between women and men in this context are also representative of the changing nature of gender roles in British society more generally as traditional roles continue to be publicly and privately both reinforced and challenged (Reed 2006). Annandale (2009) has argued that we are living through a period of striking gender-related social change in the West as traditional distinctions between women and men are breaking down and being reconfigured in new, more complex ways. Furthermore, Annandale and Hunt (2000) also argue that the contemporary social relations of gender belie easily a summary in terms of losses and gains on the part of either women or men. They argue that gender relations have changed to include new and more complex forms of equality and inequality for both men and women. They identify several key areas of social life within which traditional gender patterns are changing – the family and household, education and employment. The gender roles occupied by both women and men within this study, as will be shown within this section, in many ways reflect broader gender-related changes identified across the public and private realm.

Annandale and Hunt (2000) identify the domestic realm as an area of significant change. This includes changes in the gendering of housework and childcare. Authors such as Giddens (1992) have emphasised the democratising transformation of intimacy, leading towards a more equal set of gender relations in the domestic realm. However, many others have argued that there is little change in the domestic realm in relation to previously gendered tasks. Jackson (2008) splits domestic work into housework and childcare and concludes that there are both losses and gains here. She argues that although men are now more involved in childcare, domestic work still falls largely to women (Jackson 2008). However, as shown throughout this book and by other authors, men's increased involvement in parenting is not necessarily straightforward. For example Hanuari and Hollingworth (2009) conducted a study funded by the Joseph Rowntree foundation on fatherhood, masculinity, diversity and change in modern Britain. They found that on the surface beliefs and attitudes of fathers, mothers and children suggest that parenting roles are less strictly differentiated than they once were. They argue that it has become normal to see fathering as multi-dimensional. However, the findings of their study also revealed the persistence of some traditional gender stereotypes in practice. For example, they found that certain roles were still seen as predominantly the father's responsibility, such as financial provider, disciplinarian and involvement in leisure and play. In their study particularly economic provision still defined the father's role and ideas about 'good fathering'. Furthermore, as stated earlier a number of authors have argued that while it is true that cultural understandings of both fatherhood and masculinity are diverse and changing (Lupton and Barclay 1997, Wall and Arnold 2007), it is also the case that involved fathering continues to clash with hegemonic cultural ideals of masculinity (Connell 2000). Brandth and Kvande (1998) further reinforce this argument in their study on stay-at-home dads. They show that the domains of pregnancy, childcare and housework continue to be gendered in a traditionally feminine way which inhibits men who want to cross this boundary. Certainly the findings of this study on gender and prenatal screening tended to reflect precisely this, men were more involved in pregnancy and screening but often in ways perhaps that were not perceived to pose a direct threat to a traditional sense of masculinity.

As argued earlier, Lorber (1994) has stated that inequality between men and women is often reduced to sexual difference. However, she argues that it is the institutions of gender that lead to inequality. In particular, she highlights women's lack of rights in the public realm as playing a key role in their positions of subordination in both public and private realms. However, if we shift our focus from the private to public realm we see similar complex changes in the social relations of gender taking place. For example, as Ringrose and Epstein (2008) argue girls have been outperforming boys in education in the UK from the 1990s onwards. However, this success is often placed in contrast to a prevailing discourse around failing boys, thus leading to gender reverse binaries and anxieties (Ringrose and Epstein 2008). Furthermore, throughout the book we have explored the ways in which men's association with paid work often prevented their full involvement with their partner's pregnancy and antenatal care. However, women's persistent association with pregnancy, childcare and domestic work continues to disadvantage them in the labour market.

Irving (2008) for example highlights the complexities of contemporary patterns of gender and employment. In 1971 women accounted for just over a third of those employed. In contrast, recent statistics in the UK show women's participation rate at 69.9 per cent is slightly higher than the US (69.2) (OECD 2005). However, as Irving (2008) argues this increased participation of women in the labour market does not necessarily imply that their presence is accepted, valued or rewarded in the same way as that of men. Most women are disproportionately found in low paying occupations, and in lower status jobs in more highly paid occupations, along with lower pay (Irving 2008). As argued earlier, this model of gender and work supports the idea of men as the 'unencumbered worker' free from caring and domestic duties (Hochschild 1989, 2001, Crompton 2006), in contrast to the 'woman worker' associated with part-time low status work, the domestic sphere and childcare (Scott 2006, Halrynjo 2009). Therefore the gender paradoxes highlighted through the findings of this study on prenatal screening are merely a reflection of broader patterns of gender equality and inequalities in both the private and public realm.

In evaluating gender roles and inequalities in gender Walby (1990) developed distinctions between external and internal forms of patriarchy. She argued that British society has shifted in form from a 'private' (domestic) to 'public' patriarchy. This according to her signals a decrease in domestic work for women and an increase in educational opportunity leading to greater equality for some women and men. However, she argues that this also leads to greater segregation between women. This is because segregation is at the heart of public patriarchy, as women are drawn into the public domain but segregated within it (Walby 1990). Two issues can be noted here in relation to the findings of this study on screening. As shown throughout the book, men certainly take on more roles during pregnancy alleviating women of some of the previous burdens of the domestic realm. However, the increasing use of prenatal technology as part of a routine programme of antenatal care exemplifies a broader shift in the experience of pregnancy: from one which has historically taken place predominantly in the private realm to one which has become not just increasingly medicalised[1] but also progressively public. Furthermore, it is often the institutions and organisations of gender operating in the public realm that have inhibited men's fuller participation – in both pregnancy and reproduction. Therefore in evaluating the findings of this study it cannot be said that there has been a straightforward shift perhaps from the prevalence of internal to external forms of patriarchy but rather, a displacement of private issues to the public realm.

In the context of this study and this book, we are left therefore with a final set of questions. Is men's current involvement in screening enough, are gender roles as equal as they can be, can men take more genetic responsibility? Do women and men want men to be more involved? Is this achievable through policy and practice? The final sections of this chapter therefore will be devoted to exploring whether men can and should be more involved in screening and if so how. These issues will be explored firstly through accounts from respondents and secondly through a focus on policy, professional and ideological issues required for change.

Could men matter more? Enhancing male participation

At the end of each interview both male and female respondents within this study were asked whether they would like men to be more involved in screening. If so, how did they think men's roles could be enhanced? Most respondents coveted an increase in male involvement. Many women did want their partners to be more involved than they currently were. This can be seen in Rosie's account below. Rosie was in the second trimester of pregnancy:

INTERVIEWER: Why would you like him to be more involved? Is there any particular reason?

ROSIE: Just so he knows what's going on, so I don't have to do everything on my own, because when I go (to clinic) I can't really remember everything.

(Rosie, 27, Housewife)

When asked, many men also indicated that they would like to be more involved in their partners' screening. As Bill states: 'Given the chance I would like to be more involved. You know, I'd like to know more what's going on, what's happening to her (partner) and at what point (in the pregnancy) and that' (Bill, 37, Electrician).

Some women within the study felt that men should be able to be more involved in pregnancy and screening, and that they should take greater responsibility in the domestic realm more generally. Women sometimes felt men could do more around the house during their pregnancy. This perhaps resonates with arguments made earlier by others on men's limited advances in domestic work (Jackson 2008). Female respondents in this study also discussed ways in which antenatal care could be better organised to include men and encourage male participation. Rebecca for example who was in the second trimester of pregnancy discussed greater flexibility in antenatal appointments as a way to enable men's greater involvement:

INTERVIEWER: I don't want to hold you up because I know you've got to get going, but do you think that men should be more involved, or less?

REBECCA: They should be more involved.

INTERVIEWER: In what ways?

REBECCA: They should have the option to attend all appointments with me, they should do what they can to help you out around the house, things like that. They should help with older children. We take on all the responsibility of carrying the child, they should do their bit where they can.

(Rebecca, 36, Housewife)

This request for greater flexibility in antenatal appointments was emphasised by both female and male respondents. For example, as can be seen in the accounts from Suzie's partner Ben:

> Well, I wish they had appointments after work that would help a lot, it would be much easier to go with her. I don't see why they can't, you know, you can get a late GP appointment in our surgery, why not midwife? Midwife appointments always seem to be in the mornings, it's not fair.
>
> (Ben, 34, Customer support technician)

As shown throughout the book, one of the main constraints on men's involvement in the study was their inability to get time off work to attend appointments. Men often felt that employers were quite inflexible when it came to letting them have time off to attend partners' screening appointments.

Along with greater flexibility in appointment times therefore respondents also felt that greater flexibility in men's actual work would also aid their involvement. This can be seen in accounts from both women and men:

> Well, his work needs to let him off more to come with me. At the minute he often has to take holiday if he wants to be involved. He should be able to take time off anyway to come along.
>
> (Suzie, 34, Housewife)

> I wish I could get more time off work without having to think about the financial consequences. Men need more help in that direction. More entitlements, employers could be a bit more caring.
>
> (Alan, 40, Plumber)

In trying to improve men's involvement in screening one of the other issues raised by respondents was that of information. As argued in Chapter 1, many respondents felt that information was directed specifically to women – although men were now accessing more pregnancy-related information on the Internet. Some respondents (although at times cynical about increasing men's involvement) did feel that in order to aide men's participation, health professionals could direct more information to men. Respondents discussed two ways of doing this: directing leaflets at men and getting men to attend antenatal classes. This can be seen in the account from Emily who was in the second trimester of pregnancy:

> Erm, I don't know. I mean you could have more classes and information directed at them, I think a lot of them (men) sort of have an aversion to going to classes on pregnancy and things, dragging them along to antenatal classes and stuff like that. It isn't always a good experience for them (men). They don't get much out of – well some men do – but a lot of men say 'I don't really want to go to this', so I don't know ... but they (midwives) could encourage men more ... give them more information on what's going on. ... so at least they (men) can *feel* part of it.
>
> (Emily, 30, Health professional)

Other women felt that more antenatal or parenting classes would help men become more involved in screening and pregnancy. Flo, who was in the third trimester of pregnancy, raised this issue. She felt that although her partner Paul was very involved in her pregnancy and screening, this could be enhanced further by more parenting groups directed at men:

INTERVIEWER: Do you think its right that men have a sort of equal role, well, as equal as possible?

FLO: Yeah, I mean yeah if you're in sort of relationship then you make decisions together

INTERVIEWER: You're co-parenting.
ANGE: Yeah, I mean there's nothing that I do that Mark hasn't done, apart from the risky bit.
INTERVIEWER: You mean give birth! Do you think there are other ways that their involvement could be enhanced?
FLO: I think there should be parenting groups for men.
(Flo, 35, Self-employed)

Eleanor who was in the third trimester of pregnancy discussed a couple of ways in which men could become more involved in the process. She found antenatal classes really useful for opening her partner's eyes to pregnancy and screening. However, in the context of the health trust where this study was based, antenatal classes came quite late on in the pregnancy and focused on labour and the postnatal period. She felt that perhaps some kind of direct meeting between men and midwives or a lecture at the start of pregnancy might help men be more involved in screening.

> Yeah, I mean we did the antenatal classes at the maternity hospital, which I must say, before we did that he hadn't got a clue what was going on, and that really opened his eyes. So maybe something like, some kind of lecture thing at the beginning (of routine antenatal care), you know? I don't know. I don't know. Apart from a system that maybe they (men) come to a couple of meetings with a midwife. Maybe at twelve weeks and twenty five weeks or something, I don't know. I don't know what else you could do really. I mean you could do leaflets or whatever, but I don't know whether that would work.
> (Eleanor, 34, Director of family company)

A number of women and men within the study wanted to enhance men's involvement in the process of screening and suggested concrete ways in which men could be more involved. As shown here these related broadly to four issues: to greater flexibility in the scheduling of antenatal appointments (both hospital and community), to greater employer flexibility to enable men time off work to attend appointments, to directing more pregnancy-related information directly to men, and finally to enhancing male contact with health professionals through antenatal classes and meetings with midwives. However, although respondents often wanted men as involved as possible, they also recognised the limits to this involvement.

Limits to men's involvement

Many respondents wanted men to be more involved in prenatal screening. However, some were less bothered and others recognised that this was not always possible. Furthermore, some respondents felt that men should not be pushed into being involved. This can be seen in the accounts from one respondent, Lucy who was in the second trimester of her pregnancy. She felt that men should not be pressured to be involved because their social circumstances may not always allow participation:

> I think that men that do come along are probably quite welcome ... But it's very difficult isn't it because so many people work these days. It's difficult to get time of work and I'm quite fortunate that William is quite flexible, so generally he can come along to things. But a lot of men can't do that and it's a shame to put undue pressure on people as you don't want to go the other way and make men feel guilty.
>
> (Lucy, 35, Hospital doctor)

A few women felt that there was simply no way for men to be more involved, that actually men were in fact as involved in the process as they could possibly be. This can be seen in the account from Christine who was in the third trimester of pregnancy.

INTERVIEWER: Would you have liked him to have been more involved?
CHRISTINE: I don't think he could have been really. I mean these blood tests were routine, but he went to all the scans, and we had the twenty week growth scan, which they didn't have last time.

(Christine, 34, IT consultant)

Christine related the difficulty of getting men more involved to the differences in men and women's roles in reproduction. She related this difference to the materiality of pregnancy as discussed in the introduction to this book. She felt that as pregnancy takes place in women's bodies and is part of their biology it is obvious that they were more involved than men. She felt that men on the other hand are physically distant from this process and therefore often the experience of pregnancy is literately quite alien for them.

CHRISTINE: Yeah, I don't know. I suppose if they're not interested, they're not interested. You can give them a picture (from fetal ultrasound scan) and get 'eugh?'
INTERVIEWER: Could you get them to be more involved perhaps?
CHRISTINE: I don't know ... when she (baby) kicks and it's like come on, put your hand there, and it's just not the same.
INTERVIEWER: Not the same as feeling it?
CHRISTINE: No, no. And they're (men) just like watching telly and you're like, feel it, feel it! And they're like what?

(Christine, 34, IT consultant)

This reinforces the argument made earlier about the ways in which men's roles as genetic inseminators, present at conception, are often distanced in time and space from the material realities of pregnancy and child birth

(Sandelowski 1994). Christine was not the only respondent to reduce the differences in participation down to physiological differences between women and men. Other female respondents also highlighted the importance of the corporeal reality of pregnancy – that women's role is more important simply because pregnancy takes place in women's bodies. Kerry talked about men's participation being related to individual choice; however, she also positions this against the materiality of pregnancy taking place in women's bodies.

INTERVIEWER: And do you think overall, should men be more or less involved?

KERRY: I suppose it depends on the individual doesn't it? I mean I'm lucky that my husband wants to play a part. So I don't know how important it is for the man, it's the women who are actually being pregnant and having to do it.

INTERVIEWER: And do you think there's any way the man's role could be enhanced, or if it's not necessary in the screening processes?

KERRY: Not really, because I don't really see them as *so* [strong emphasis] important.

(Kerry, 29, Housewife)

While some respondents raised the issue of the material limits to men's participation, in pregnancy and screening others however felt that it was just hard to get men interested in 'women's' concerns such as pregnancy and childbirth. This reaffirms the argument made by other authors such as Rapp (2000) in that many men feel that pregnancy is a woman's domain. This can be seen in Suzie's account below:

> I don't know, and sometimes it does make you feel like you're wringing them (men) out. But there isn't actually a way that I could get him more involved, and with the screening and the scans and things like that, there's only two occasions when you go there (hospital clinic). And they're quite early on, so the other twenty weeks or however long you actually are pregnant for, I don't know, it's sort of lost time really. When they (men) notice that your tummy's getting bigger and then they can feel the baby kick, that helps, but apart from that … what can you do?
>
> (Suzie, 34, Housewife)

This respondent did want her partner to be more involved but felt that she almost had to force him to be more involved by constantly thrusting pregnancy information at him. She also felt that the daily grind of work and existing childcare commitments often placed constraints on men's greater involvement.

INTERVIEWER: Overall how did you feel about his involvement?

SUZIE: Erm, I think there could be more of an involvement, definitely. But I don't know how. I don't know what could happen to get him more

> involved. I think it's probably a personal thing between the couple in the relationship, there's nothing else that anyone could do to get him more involved, it's between yourselves. I've sort of stuck pregnancy magazines under his nose and said oh, look at that. Because they do have Dad's sections, and stuff like that in magazines, but I don't know. It's sort of like, we've already got a child as well, who's six, so you know, and with his school work and doing out of hours activities with him (existing child), we don't always get enough time to do anything else ... And plus with working as well, I didn't finish work till a couple of weeks ago, so we were both at work all day and then at night, you know after tea and bath time and bed time and you finally sit down. Then there are other things to discuss like what's happened that day, rather than read this article about what Dad's (to be) should be doing.
>
> (Suzie, 34, Housewife)

Whilst recognising that there were limits – both biological and social – to men's involvement in pregnancy screening, most respondents did nonetheless want men to be involved. There was only one respondent in the study who was particularly ambivalent to enhancing her partner's participation. This was Emma who was in the second trimester of pregnancy:

INTERVIEWER: Would you want him to be more involved?

EMMA: No not at all. Even if (he) were less (involved) I'd be alright. I know what men are like and some of them aren't that bothered. It wouldn't really bother me because I expect him to be. It's not that he doesn't care it's just that it's not his thing, but I'd be ok if he wasn't as assertive you know, as long as he asked if I was alright and stuff like that.

(Emma, 22, Nanny)

Both male and female respondents often articulated a desire for men to be more involved in screening but felt that they shouldn't be pressured; it should be left to the individual couple. In terms of enabling men's greater involvement some women and men identified organisational and institutional changes which could foster greater involvement. However, while most women wanted men to be more involved, what also came across was women's desire for ultimate control over their pregnancies and bodies. In the final section of the book therefore, the practical and ideological potential for enabling men's increased involvement in screening will be explored, along with the recognition of maintaining women's reproductive autonomy.

Gender and prenatal screening: constraints and possible future roles

This book has highlighted the importance of men's involvement in prenatal blood screening, whilst also emphasising the continued need for women's reproductive autonomy. While the book has raised some important issues relating to gender roles in screening it is important to acknowledge its limitations. The study on which the book is based was small scale and therefore it is important not to generalise from the findings of the study. Furthermore, most of the respondents within the study received 'normal' screening results. Where they did receive 'risky' screening results and had further screening or took part in diagnostic testing, all respondents went on to have 'normal' pregnancies. Therefore the book cannot speak for couples who have entered the realm of prenatal diagnosis and selective abortion. While recognising the limitations of such a small-scale study, the book has raised the importance of men's roles in prenatal blood screening along with the barriers to their involvement.

Drawing on a broad array of research findings on men's roles in pregnancy and fatherhood across Europe, the WHO (2007) has concluded that the increased involvement by fathers during pregnancy can positively affect health outcomes for men, their partners and children. Despite this, however, they also argue that the maternal and child health services in Europe still have difficulties in attracting and increasing the roles of fathers in official parenting and antenatal programmes (Plantin 2001). Even if men attend programmes, they often feel marginalised and not directly addressed by the staff (Finnbogadottir *et al.* 2003). This means that men generally get less information and are often less prepared for parenting. Maternal and childcare programmes have also had particular difficulty in reaching certain groups of parents and fathers, for example, immigrant fathers, and fathers on low incomes and adolescent fathers (Schott and Henley 1997). Largely speaking within this study both men and women would like men to have been more involved in their partner's prenatal care, including further participation in screening. However, both men and women often felt that social and institutional barriers prevented them from doing so – in particular health professionals and workplace norms. In light of these constraints a number of tentative suggestions can be made to enable men's greater involvement.

Changes in professional practice

The UK screening commission gives clear guidelines to midwives when it comes to male participation in screening decision-making. It emphasises the need for practitioners to recognise the importance of women's reproductive autonomy whilst at the same time where possible encouraging men's involvement (UK National Screening Committee 2007). Despite this emphasis, however, many male respondents interviewed within the study felt that health professionals 'pushed them out' of their partners' screening experiences, making screening a 'woman only' affair (Reed 2011a). As argued earlier, this resonates with the findings of other studies which highlight the ways in which men are regularly dismissed in antenatal consultations and seldom approached directly by the midwife (Olsson and Jansson 2001). Men often feel that they are not made to feel welcome by midwives in the female-dominated environment of the antenatal clinic. Midwives' main aim is to protect women's reproductive autonomy in this context. However, in excluding men they are also systematically reinforcing the traditionally gendered nature of reproduction. As stated earlier Vosler and Burst (1993) argue that midwives both uphold and transform traditional gender roles within prenatal care. According to them, this relates to the fact that midwives are a profession of women, serving the health needs of women in a health care system that has been historically dominated by men. Midwives try to work in the interests of the women they serve whilst also being constrained by a medical system which continues to reinforce a traditional gender division of labour in the reproductive sphere (Reed 2011a).

Respondents' accounts often articulated a desire for midwives to encourage male participation, for men to be addressed more directly by them during antenatal consultations. In light of this in future perhaps midwives and health practitioners working within prenatal clinics could perhaps take more consideration of the importance of men's roles (Reed 2011a). This would mean including men more fully in screening consultation, providing more information specifically for men, having greater flexibility in appointment times, and generally making men feel more welcome during the process. As already acknowledged, midwives are undoubtedly in a difficult position in the prenatal clinic. They must encourage male participation whilst also ensuring women's reproductive choice and autonomy, all within the context of a highly pressurised screening environment where they may have multiple obligations, to women, to their employer, to colleagues and various other agencies (Levy 1999; Markens, Browner and Preloran 2003). It is essential therefore that we consider the workload implications for midwives and genetic counsellors resulting from any enhancement of men's existing roles. As the Human Genetics Commission report (2005) highlights, the screening environment is a highly pressurised one where staff are dealing with more cases then there is often capacity for. Therefore health professionals need to be consulted on any potential increase in men's roles (Reed 2011a).

Changes in employment policy and legislation

One of the key issues preventing men's involvement in their partner's antenatal care in this study related to men's inability to get time off work. Unsurprising therefore greater work flexibility was emphasised in respondents' accounts as a way of enhancing men's involvement in the future. Changes in government legislation enabling men to take time off work for their partner's screening appointments without incurring financial penalties or using annual leave would enable men's greater participation. This would be particularly beneficial to men in unskilled and semi-skilled employment who often find it difficult to take time off to attend their partner's screening appointments. Coupled together these changes would enable men to engage more fully with the experience of pregnancy and to heighten their roles and responsibilities as potential fathers.

The practical implications of improving employer flexibility undoubtedly require further investigation. The cost of so-called family friendly policies in the work place has already been given some consideration. Employers have identified both advantages and disadvantages of policies such as flexible working hours, paternity leave, etc. – on the one hand they are seen to boost staff morale, on the other hand they place an increasing administrative burden on employers (Forth *et al.* 1997). Despite this, significant changes have taken place regarding paid paternity leave in the UK. From April 2011, some men in the UK will be entitled to additional paid paternity leave. This is based on a shared model of parental leave after childbirth (Direct.gov.uk 2011). While the issue of longer and paid paternity leave has received recent attention in the UK, the specific implications of men's involvement in prenatal appointments, still needs greater consideration. As argued earlier, within the UK there is no legislation as yet that allows men the legal right to take time off work to attend their partners' screening appointments (Fatherhood Institute 2004). The government has produced a 'Good Practice' leaflet for employers. This leaflet highlights the importance of men's attendance at their partner's screening. However, it emphasises that screening appointment times cannot be changed to be more accommodating as: 'There is little flexibility in when these appointments can be held, as midwives will be caring for a number of expectant women' (Department of Trade and Industry 2004: 5). However, it does encourage employers to enable male workers time off to attend screening (Department of Trade and Industry 2004). However, whether they do or not remains at the discretion of individual employers.

Reproductive autonomy, responsibility and choice

The issue of women's reproductive choice must also not be forgotten here. Despite their desire for increased male involvement what was very clear in the accounts of female respondents in this study was the need for women to maintain ultimate control over reproductive decision-making. As argued throughout the book women's rights to make decisions over their reproductive health has been a long fought battle which has been central to feminist debates over the last few decades (Markens, Browner and Preloran 2003). The issue of women's reproductive autonomy and choice has remained at the centre of much feminist work on NRTs (Petchesky 1984; Corea 1985). There is therefore a need to increase men's roles but continue to place women's autonomy at the centre of screening decision-making.

Women in this study articulated an overall positive experience of male involvement in antenatal care. However, other studies have shown that this is not always the case. For example, in a study on pregnancy and domestic violence by Stenson *et al.* (2005), it was found that when men were present during prenatal consultations there were often problems with male partners dominating the conversations, answering for the woman, making the decisions and acting as an interpreter. In cases such as these it may be preferable for men not to be involved. To go back to my own experiences of antenatal care articulated in the introduction, one of the first things my community midwife did at her initial home visit with me was to send my husband upstairs. She did this so that she could give me a minuscule leaflet in private on domestic violence in pregnancy. When I asked why the leaflet was so small, she said it was small enough to fit in a woman's sock so that women could (if necessary) hide it from potentially violent husbands. Male bullying in pregnancy therefore is a very real problem that should not be underestimated in enhancing men's participation. This emphasises the need to continue to place 'choice' at the centre of any screening consultation (Markens, Browner and Preloran 2003). This refers both to women's reproductive choice and autonomy and also to men's choice. As articulated by one of the respondents (Lucy) earlier in this chapter, while encouraging male involvement, we do not want to get to a position where men feel browbeaten by health professionals and women into participation. Their participation in screening has to be perceived to be beneficial to all involved (Reed 2011a).

Beyond gender and (genetics)

Finally, we have addressed potential changes made to screening practice and to government legislation on men's involvement. However, what about the gendered nature of genetics and gender role ideology? Undoubtedly, men's ability to be involved in screening will continue to be limited by biology; unless they are participants of screening themselves men's roles will be somewhat curtailed. In the small number of cases within this study where men were also recipients of screening, there did actually seem to be a more of a shift towards equal gender roles (Reed 2009). This sharing of genetics through male screening has the potential to challenge the materiality of pregnancy. In these cases the 50/50 contribution of hereditary materials appears to challenge pre-existing gendered nature of genetics. However, men's sharing in the corporeality of pregnancy is unusual and only happens when women test positive for inherited blood disorders. The equal gendering of genetics therefore is only likely to affect a small minority of couples. Where men are not materially involved in screening, traditionally gendered associations of reproduction and genetic contributions while less pronounced continue at some level to persist. Simply put this relates directly to the fact that pregnancy takes place in women's not men's bodies. Therefore the visceral effects of the process continue to be more keenly felt by women (Dragonas 2001).

Despite these material constraints to gender and reproduction, however, gender role ideology continues to play a powerful role. Reflecting back on discussions outlined in the introduction around the issue of theorising gender in the contemporary world, it is important to acknowledge (as many others have) that the social relations of gender are fluid, multiple and continually subject to change (Annandale and Hunt 2000; Francis 2008). However, gender role ideology in my view does continue to influence the positions women and men adopt at particular points in time. In the context of this study as articulated, it continues to reinforce men's peripheral role in their partners' screening through associating women with child bearing and men with paid work. Through reinforcing the starkly gendered nature of reproduction this ideology has the potential to hinder individual men's involvement in screening. It also places constraints on the possibility of institutional and organisational change. If men continue to be associated with paid work and women with reproduction then there will be no impetus for health professionals or employers to encourage, facilitate or enable men's greater involvement. Fortunately, as the data from this and other studies on prenatal screening show, there is evidence to suggest that the desire for men's involvement in screening is greater than the desire for the maintenance of traditional gender roles (Reed 2011a). With this in mind we can start to implement change to support men's participation in screening at an institutional and organisational level and ideological change, although gradual, should follow. As Lorber (1994) has argued, gender has changed in the past and will change in the future. However, without deliberate restructuring it will not necessarily change towards greater gender equality between women and men. Making various organisational and institutional changes in the prenatal arena will hopefully lead towards greater equality and responsibility for both parents.

Appendix

Table A.1 Summary of pregnant women

Name	*Pregnancy number*	*Trimester*	*Age*	*Marital status*	*Ethnicity*	*Occupation*	*Religion*
Kerry	2nd	2	29	Cohabiting	White British	Housewife	None
Emily	2nd	2	30	Cohabiting	White British	Health professional	None
Rebecca	3rd	2	36	Cohabiting	White British	Housewife	None
Suzie	2nd	2	34	Cohabiting	White British	Housewife	None
Linda	3rd	3	30	Cohabiting	White British	Child minder	None
Rosie	5th	2	27	Cohabiting	White British	Housewife	None
Zoe	1st	3	31	Married	White British	Museum's officer	Agnostic
Liz	1st	3	32	Married	White British	University researcher	Catholic
Kylie	1st	2	28	Married	White British	Nurse	Christian
Emma	1st	2	22	Cohabiting	White British	Nanny	Catholic
Jan	1st	1	32	Married	British Asian	Hairdresser	None
Sarah	1st	2	33	Married	White British	Teacher	None
Pinky	1st	2	30	Married	British Asian	Bank clerk	Hindu
Flo	2nd	3	35	Cohabiting	British Mauritian	Self-employed	None
Eleanor	2nd	3	34	Married	White British	Director of family company	Church of England
Katarina	1st	1	28	Married	Czech	Self-employed	Christian
Joanne	1st	2	35	Married	White British	Nurse	None
Christine	2nd	3	34	Married	White British	IT consultant	None
Chelsea	1st	3	25	Married	White British	Care worker	None
Jameela	1st	3	37	Cohabiting	African	Student accountant	Muslim
Trish	1st	2	38	Cohabiting	White British	Academic	None
Lucy	1st	2	35	Married	White British	Hospital doctor	None

Table A.2 Summary of male partners

Name	*Age*	*Partner*	*Occupation*	*Ethnicity*	*Religion*
Bill	37	Rebecca	Electrician	White British	None
John	37	Christine	Currently unemployed	White British	None
William	35	Lucy	GP	White British	None
Paul	31	Paul	Self-employed	White British	None
Morris	37	Trish	Artist	White British	None
Rob	25	Chelsea	Factory worker	White British	None
Keith	35	Joanne	Artist	White British	None
Pete	31	Rosie	Plasterer	White British	None
Dave	31	Zoe	Graphic designer	White British	None
Brendan	33	Liz	Travel agent	White Irish	Catholic
Sean	30	Kylie	Self-employed	White Irish	Christian
Bihar	31	Pinky	Shop owner	South Asian	Hindu
Tunde	37	Jameela	Psychiatrist	Black African	Muslim
Alan	40	Jan	Plumber	White British	None
Nick	32	Sarah	Teacher	White British	None
Ben	34	Suzie	Customer support technician	White British	None

Notes

Introduction

1 For a thorough discussion of the concept of patriarchy see Walby, S. (1990) *Theorizing Patriarchy,* Oxford: Blackwell.
2 Although not directly inherited, there are a small number of cases where a woman's chance of having more than one baby with Down's syndrome is increased. This occurs when Down's syndrome develops due to chromosomal translocations (this accounts for around 4 per cent of cases). This process involves the transfer of part of one chromosome to another and may reflect an abnormal chromosome arrangement in one of the parents. If this is the case the chance of a further child having Down's syndrome is significantly increased (see NHS Evidence (a) (accessed 2011) for further information).
3 For a full discussion on ethics procedures in health-related research, refer to Reed (2007a).
4 An abridged version of *The National Statistics Socio-Economic Classification* (NS-SEC) classificatory system was used to situate respondents into occupational categories. [www.statistics.gov.uk/methods_quality/ns_sec/] (accessed 2009).
5 The Mauritian respondent was of Indian descent.
6 Women in the study sometimes referred to male partners by name even though these men were not interviewed as part of the study. While these names may appear in the main text, the summary of male respondents in the appendix relates only to direct participants in the study.

3 Imaging and imagining genetics

1 See NHS Encyclopaedia for further information on Rhesus disease. www.nhsdirect.wales.nhs.uk/encyclopaedia/r/article/rhesusdisease/ (accessed 2011).

5 Gendering 'good' and 'bad' genes

1 Within the study, one couple chose not to have the triple test for religious reasons. Other couples chose not to have the test because they wanted to keep the baby regardless of any potential disability.
2 Despite respondents' more blasé views about inherited blood disorders, it is important to emphasise that both sickle cell anaemia and beta thalassaemia are serious conditions. If you have sickle cell disease, blood cells can get stuck when moving through small blood vessels, stopping the supply of oxygen to parts of your body. This often results in pain, tissue damage, and can lead to other serious complications, such as a stroke or blindness. The only cure is a bone marrow

transplant. Beta thalassaemia major affects the body's ability to create red blood cells. People with this condition often feel tired, breathless, lethargic and faint. It can also cause other complications including organ damage, restricted growth, liver disease, heart failure and death. People with beta thalassaemia major will need to receive blood transfusions all their lives. For further information see http://sct.screening.nhs.uk/ (accessed June 2011).

6 Family, friends and heredity

1 The issue of racialisation will be returned to in Chapter 7.

7 Transforming social divisions

1 *See* www.statistics.gov.uk/methods_quality/ns_sec/ (accessed 2009).
2 The term black and minority ethnic is used here to refer to people who do not identify as White British. This term can however include those who identify as minority White populations in Britain including Irish, Welsh, Scottish and those seeking Asylum (see Parliamentary Office of Science and Technology (2007) *Postnote*) for the use of BME in health policy and Research. www.parliment.uk/post
3 British whiteness is used here to refer to a majority population. This does not include those who identify as white minority populations (see above).
4 For a more thorough discussion of class and capital see Skeggs (2001).
5 Costs vary depending on hospital and also on whether a couple opts for just the nuchal scan alone or the combined or integrated tests which include both blood screening and ultrasound scanning.

Conclusion

1 The medicalisation of pregnancy has long been the subject of feminist discussions on pregnancy and child birth. There is no space to explore these particular debates in detail here. For further information see Oakley (2005).

Bibliography

Acker, J. (1990) 'Hierarchies, jobs, bodies: a theory of gendered organizations', *Gender and Society*, 4(2): 139–58.

Adam, B. (1992) 'Time and health implicated: a conceptual critique' in R. Frankenberg (ed.) *Time, Health and Medicine*, London: Sage.

Ahmad, W.I.U. and Bradby, H. (2007) 'Locating ethnicity and health: exploring concepts and contexts', *Sociology of Health and Illness*, 29(6): 795–810.

Ainsworth, S. and Cutcher, L. (2008) 'Expectant mothers and absent fathers: paid maternity leave in Australia', *Gender, Work and Organization*, 15(4): 375–93.

Allison, P. (1954) 'Protection afforded to sickle cell trait against subtertian malarial infection', *British Medical Journal*, 1: 290–94.

Annandale, E. (2009) *Women's Health and Social Change*, London: Routledge.

Annandale, E. and Clark, J. (1996) 'What is gender? Feminist theory and the sociology of human reproduction', *Sociology of Health and Illness*, 18(1): 17–44.

Annandale, E. and Hunt, K. (eds) (2000) *Gender Inequalities in Health*, Buckingham: Open University Press.

Atkin, K., Ahmad, W.I.U. and Anionwu, E.N. (1998) 'Screening and counselling for sickle cell disorders and thalassaemia: the experience of parents and health professionals', *Social Science and Medicine*, 47(11): 1639–51.

Austrin, T. and Farnsworth, J. (2005) 'Hybrid genes: fieldwork, detection and the method of Bruno Latour', *Qualitative Research*, 5(2): 147–65.

Babay, Z. (2004) 'Attitudes of a high-risk group of pregnant Saudi Arabian women to prenatal screening for chromosomal anomalies', *Eastern Mediterranean Health Journal*, 10(4/5): 522–7.

Babycentre UK www.babycentre.co.uk/ (accessed February 2011).

Baillie, C., Smith, J., Hewison, J. and Mason, G. (2000) 'Ultrasound screening for fetal abnormality: women's reactions to false positive results', *British Journal of Health Psychology*, 5: 377–94.

Barclay, L. and Lupton, D. (1999) 'The experiences of new fatherhood: a socio-cultural analysis', *Journal of Advanced Nursing*, 29(4): 1013–20.

Barnes, L. and Boddy, J. (1994) *Aman, the Story of a Somali Girl*, London: Bloomsbury.

Bartlett, E. (2004) 'The effects of fatherhood on the health of men: a review of the literature', *The Journal of Men's Health and Gender*, 1(2–3): 159–69.

BBC News (2008) 'Many keeping babies with Down's' (24/11/2008) http://news.bbc.co.uk/1/hi/health/7741411.stm (accessed June 2011).

Beck, U. (1992) *Risk Society: Towards a New Modernity*, New Delhi: Sage.

Berry, L. (1988) 'Realistic expectations of the labour coach', *Journal of Obstetric, Gynecologic and Neonatal Nursing*, 17: 354–5.

Bourdieu, P. (1979) *Distinction: A Social Critique of the Judgment of Taste*, trans. Richard Nice, 1984. Boston, USA: Harvard University Press.

Bowler, I. (1993) 'They're not the same as us: midwives' stereotypes of South Asian descent maternity patients', *Sociology of Health and Illness*, 15(2): 157–78.

Brandth, B. and Kvande, K. (1998) 'Masculinity and fathering: the reconstruction of childcare', *Sociological Review*, 46(2): 293–313.

Brett, K., Schoendorf, K.C. and Kiely, J.L. (1994) 'Differences between black and white women's use of prenatal care technologies', *American Journal of Obstetrics and Gynecology*, 170(1): 41–6.

Browner, C. H., Preloran, M. and Cox, S. (1999) 'Ethnicity, bioethics and prenatal diagnosis: the amniocentesis decisions of Mexican-origin women and their partners', *Public Health Matters*, 89(11): 1658–66.

Bryman, A. (2001) *Social Research Methods*, Oxford: Oxford University Press.

Bunting, M. (2004) *Willing Slaves: How the Overwork Culture is Ruling Our Lives* London: Harper Collins.

Cannon, L.W., Higgenbotham, E. and Leung, M.L.A. (1988) 'Race and class bias in qualitative research on women', *Gender and Society*, 2: 449–62.

Carroll, J.C., Brown, J.B., Reid, A.J. and Pugh, P. (2000) 'Women's experience of maternal serum screening', *Canadian Family Physician*, 46: 614–20.

Chattopadhyay, S. (2006) 'Rakter dosh-corrupting blood: the challenges of preventing thalassemia in Bengal, India', *Social Science and Medicine,* 63: 2661–73.

Chronholm, A. (2004) '*Dad on Parental Leave. Men's Experience with Shared Parental Leave'*, Göteborg, University of Göteborg, Department of Sociology.

Clarke, J. (1983) 'Sexism, feminism and medicalism: a decade review of literature on gender and illness', *Sociology of Health and Illness*, 5(1): 62–82.

Clement, S. (ed) (1998) *Psychological Perspectives on Pregnancy and Childbirth*, New York: Churchill Livingstone.

Connell, R. (2000) *The Men and the Boys*, Berkeley: University of California Press.

Conrad, P. and Gabe, J. (1999) 'Introduction: sociological perspectives on the new genetics: an overview', *Sociology of Health & Illness*, 21(5): 505–16.

Conrad, P. (1994) Presentation to the Society for the Study of Social Problems, Annual Meeting.

Conrad, P. (1997) 'Public eyes and private genes: historical frames, new constructions and social problems', *Social Problems*, 44(2): 139–54.

Corea, C. (1985) *The Mother Machine: Reproductive Technologies from Artificial Insemination to the Artificial Womb*, New York: Harper and Row.

Courtenay, W.H. (2000) 'Constructions of masculinity and their influence on men's well-being: A theory of gender and health', *Social Science & Medicine*, 50(10): 1385–401.

Craig, L. (2006) 'Does father care mean fathers share? A comparison of how mothers and fathers in intact families spend time with their children', *Gender & Society*, 20: 259–81.

Crompton, R. (2006) *Employment and the Family. The Reconfiguration of Work and Family Life in Contemporary Societies*, Cambridge: Cambridge University Press.

Crompton, R., Brockman, M. and Lyonette, C. (2005) 'Attitudes, women's employment and the domestic division of labour', *Work, Employment and Society*, 19(2): 213–33.

Delphy, C. (1992) 'Mothers' union?', *Trouble and Strife*, 24: 12–19.

Delvaux, T., Buekens, P., Godin, I. and Boutsen, M. (2001) 'Barriers to prenatal care in Europe', *American Journal of Preventative Medicine*, 21(1): 52–9.

Department of Health (1998) *Our Healthier Nation: A Contract for Health*, London: The Stationery Office.

——(2000) Second Report of the UK National Screening Committee.

——(2006) *The Pregnancy Book*, London: Central Office of Information.

Department of Trade and Industry (DTI) (2004) *Fathers-to-be and Prenatal Appointments: A Good Practice Guide.* First published November 2004, www.dti.gov.uk/ (accessed September 2008).

Dex, S. (2003) *Families and Work in the Twenty-First Century*, Bristol: The Policy Press.

Diemer, G.A. (1997) 'Expectant fathers: influence of perinatal education on stress, coping and spousal relations', *Research in Nursing and Health*, 20: 281–93.

Directgov (2011) 'Additional paternity-leave and pay' www.direct.gov.uk/ (accessed May 2011).

Down's Syndrome Association 'Stories on T.V' www.downs-syndrome.org.uk/information/i-have-downs-syndrome/eastenders.html (accessed May 2011).

Doyle, J.A. (1995) *The Male Experience*, Madison, WI: Brown and Benchmark.

Dragonas, T. (2001) 'Whose fault is it? Shame and guilt for the genetic defect', in E. Ettorre (ed), *Before Birth*, London: Ashgate.

Draper, J. (2002) 'It was a real good show': the ultrasound scan, fathers and the power of visual knowledge', *Sociology of Health & Illness*, 24(6): 771–95.

Dudgeon, M. and Inhorn, M. (2004) 'Men's influences on women's reproductive health: medical anthropological perspectives', *Social Science and Medicine*, 59: 1379–95.

Dunn, C.L., Pirie, P.L. and Hellerstedt, W.L. (2003) 'The advice-giving role of female friends and relatives during pregnancy', *Health Education Research*, 18(3): 352–62.

Duster, T. (1990) *Backdoor to Eugenics*, London: Routledge.

Dyson, S. (1999) 'Genetic screening and ethnic minorities', *Critical Social Policy*, 19 (2): 195–215.

Dyson, S., Fielder, A. and Kirkham, M. (1995) 'Haemoglobinopathies, antenatal screening and the midwife', *British Journal of Midwifery*, 4(6): 319–22.

Early, R. (2001) 'Men as consumers of maternity services: a contradiction in terms', *International Journal of Consumer Studies*, 25: 160–7.

Earle, S. and Letherby, G. (2007) 'Conceiving time? Women who do or do not conceive', *Sociology of Health & Illness*, 29(2): 233–50.

Edwards, J., Franklin, S., Hirsch, E., Price, F. and Strathern, M. (1993) *Technologies of Procreation: Kinship in the Age of Assisted Conception*, 2nd edn, London: Routledge.

Ettorre, E. (2000) 'Reproductive genetics, gender and the body: "Please doctor, may I have a normal baby?"' *Sociology*, 34(3): 403–20.

——(2002) *Reproductive Genetics, Gender and the Body*, Routledge: London.

Fatherhood Institute (2004) 'Government backs dads attending prenatal appointments' www.fatherhoodinstitute.org/index.php?id=10& cID = 31 (accessed September 2008).

Finger, A. (1990) *Past Due: A Story of Disability, Pregnancy and Childbirth*, London: The Women's Press.

Finkler, K., Skrzynia, C. and Evans, J.P. (2003) 'The new genetics and its consequences for family, kinship, medicine and medical genetics', *Social Science and Medicine*, 57: 403–12.

Finnbogadottir, H., Svalenius, E.C. and Persson, E.K. (2003) 'Expectant first-time fathers experiences of pregnancy', *Midwifery*, 19: 96–105.

Forth, J., Lissenburgh, S., Callendar, C. and Millward, N. (1997) 'Family friendly working arrangements in Britain, 1996', *Policy Studies Institute.* Department for Education and Employment. Research Brief, Number 16.

Fox-Keller, E. (1992) 'Nature, nurture and the human genome project', in D.J. Kelves and L. Hood (eds), *The Code of Codes*, Cambridge, MA: Harvard University Press.

Francis, B. (2008) 'Engendering debate: how to formulate a political account of the divide between genetic bodies and discursive gender', *Journal of Gender Studies*, 17 (3): 211–23.

Frankenberg, R. (1992) (ed.) *Time, Health and Medicine*, London: Sage.

Genome Screening Service (2007) Screening Information Leaflet www.grnomrltd.co.uk (accessed 2009).

Getz, L. and Kirkengen, A. (2003) 'Ultrasound screening in pregnancy: advanced technology, soft markers for fetal chromosomal aberrations, and unacknowledged ethical dilemmas', *Social Science and Medicine*, 56(10): 2045–57.

Giddens, A. (1981) 'Agency, institution and time-space analysis', in K. Knorr-Cetina and A.V. Cicourel (eds), *Advances in Social Theory and Methodology: Towards an Integration of Micro and Macro Sociologies*, London: Routledge.

——(1990) *The Consequences of Modernity*, Cambridge: Polity Press.

——(1991) *Modernity and Self-Identity*, Cambridge: Polity Press.

——(1992) *The Transformation of Intimacy: Sex, Love and Eroticism in Modern Societies*, Cambridge: Polity Press.

Glaser, B.G. and Strauss, A.L. (1967) *The Discovery of Grounded Theory: Strategies for Qualitative Research*, New York: Aldine.

Goldthorpe, J. (2004) *The Economic Basis of Social Class*, London: Centre for Analysis of Social Exclusion, LSE.

Good, B.J. (1994) *Medicine, Rationality and Experience: An Anthropological Perspective*, Cambridge: Cambridge University Press.

Green, J. (1995) 'Obstetricians' views on prenatal diagnosis and termination of pregnancy: 1980 compared with 1993', *British Journal of Obstetrics and Gynaecology*, 102: 228–32.

Green, J.M. (1994) 'Serum screening for Down's syndrome: experiences of obstetricians in England and Wales', *BMJ*, 309: 769–72.

Green, J.M., Hewison, J., Bekker, H.L., Bryant, L.D. and Cuckle, H.S. (2004) 'Psychosocial aspects of genetic screening of pregnant women and newborns: a systematic review', *Health Technology Assessment*, 8, 33. www.hta.ac.uk/execsumm/summ833.shtml (accessed May 2011).

Grosz, E. (1999) 'Space, time and bodies', in J. Wolmark (ed.), *Cybersexualities: A Reader on Feminist Theory, Cyborgs and Cyberspace*, Edinburgh: Edinburgh University Press.

Hall, R., Saukko, P., Evans, P.H., Qureshi, N. and Humphries, S.E. (2007) 'Assessing family history of heart disease in primary care consultations: a qualitative study', *Family Practice*, 24: 435–42.

Hallowell, N. (1999) 'Doing the right thing: genetic risk and responsibility', *Sociology of Health & Illness*, 21(5): 597–621.

Halrynjo, S. (2009) 'Men's work–life conflict: career, care and self-realization: patterns of privileges and dilemmas', *Gender, Work and Organization*, 16(1): 98–125.

Hansen, C. (2004) *A Cultural History of Pregnancy: Pregnancy Medicine and Culture 1700–2000*, Basingstoke: Palgrave.

Hardey, M. (1999) 'Doctor in the house: the internet as a source of lay health knowledge and challenge to expertise', *Sociology of Health and Illness*, 21(6): 820–35.

Haraway, D. (1991) *Simians, Cyborgs and Women: The Reinvention of Nature*, New York: Routledge.

Harris, R. and Firestone, J.M. (1998) 'Changes in predictors of gender role ideologies among women: a multivariate analysis', *Sex Roles*, 38(3–4): 239–52.

Hauari, H. and Hollingworth, K. (2009) 'Understanding fathering: masculinity, diversity and change', *Joseph Rowntree Foundation* www.jrf.org.uk/publications/understanding-fathering (accessed 2010).

Hewlett, B. (1991) *Intimate Fathers: The Nature and Context of Aka Pygmy Paternal Infant Care*, Ann Arbor, MI: University of Michigan Press.

Hindley, C., Wren Hindliff, S. and Thomson, A.M. (2006) 'English midwives views and experiences of intrapartum fetal heart rate monitoring in women at low obstetric risk: conflicts and compromises', *Journal of Midwifery and Women's Health*, 51 (5): 354–60.

Hirsch, E. (1993) 'Negotiated limits: interviews in south-east England', in J. Edwards, S. Franklin., E. Hirsch., F. Price and M. Strathern, *Technologies of Procreation: Kinship in the Age of Assisted Conception*, London: Routledge.

Hochschild, A.R. (1989) *The Second Shift*, New York: Penguin Books.

Hochschild, A.R. (2001) *The Time Bind: When Work Becomes Home and Home Becomes Work* (2nd edn first published 1997), New York, NY: Henry Holt and Company.

Hollyer, T., Boon, H., Georgousis, A., Smith, M. and Finarson, A. (2002) 'The use of CAM by women suffering from nausea and vomiting during pregnancy', *BMC Complementary and Alternative Medicine*, 2(5) www.biomedcentral.com/content/pdf/1472-6882-2-5.pdf (accessed March 2011).

Hubbard, R. (1989) 'Personal courage is not enough: some hazards of childbearing in the 1980's', in R. Arditti, R. Duelli-Klein and S. Minden (eds), *Test-Tube Women. What Future for Motherhood?* London: Pandora-Press.

Hubbard, R. (1997) 'Abortion and disability: who should and who should not inhabit the world?' In L. Davis (ed.). *The Disability Reader*, New York: Routledge.

Human Genetics Commission Committee (2002) *Inside Information: Balancing Interests in the Use of Personal Genetic Data*, London: HGC.

Human Genetics Commission Report (2005) www.hgc.gov.uk (accessed November 2005).

Innes, M. (2003) *Investigating Murder: Detective Work and the Police Response to Criminal Homicide*, Oxford: Oxford University Press.

Irving, Z. (2008) 'Gender and work', in D. Richardson and V. Robinson (eds), *Introducing Women's Studies: Feminist Theory and Practice*, 3rd edn, Basingstoke: Palgrave.

Ivry, T. (2007) 'Embodied responsibilities: pregnancy in the eyes of Japanese ob-gyns', *Sociology of Health & Illness*, 29(2): 251–74.

Jackson, A., Ervin, K., Gardner, P.D. and Schmitt, N. (2001) 'Gender and the Internet: women communicating and men searching', *Sex Roles*, 44(5/6): 363–79.

Jackson, S. (2008) 'Families, domesticity and intimacy: changing relationships in changing times', in D. Richardson and V. Robinson (eds), *Introducing Women's Studies: Feminist Theory and Practice*, 3rd edn, Basingstoke: Palgrave.

Jordan, P.L. (1990) 'Laboring for relevance: expectant and new fatherhood', *Nursing Research*, 39: 11–16.

Keller, E.F. and Grontowski, C.R. (1983) 'The mind's eye', in S. Harding and M.B. Hintikka (eds), *Discovering Reality: Feminist Perspectives on Epistemology, Metaphysics, Methodology and Philosophy of Science*, Dordrecht, Holland: D. Reidel.

Kerr, A. (2004) *Genetics and Society: A Sociology of Disease*, London: Routledge.

Kuppermann, M., Gates, E. and Washington, E. (1996) 'Racial-ethnic differences in prenatal diagnosis test use and outcomes: preferences, socioeconomics or parent knowledge?' *Obstetrics and Gynecology*, 87(5): 675–82.

Landsman, G.H. (1998) 'Reconstructing motherhood in the age of "perfect" babies: mothers of infants and toddlers with disabilities', *Signs: Journal of Women in Culture and Society*, 24(1): 9–98.

LaRossa, R. (1988) 'Fatherhood and social change', *Family Relations*, 37(4): 451–57.

LaRossa, R. (1997) *The Modernization of Fatherhood: A Social and Political History*, Chicago, IL: University of Chicago Press.

Larsson, M. (2009) 'A descriptive study of the use of the Internet by women seeking pregnancy-related information', *Midwifery*, 25: 14–20.

Lazarus, E. (1994) 'What do women want? Issues of choice, control and class in pregnancy and childbirth', *Medical Anthropology Quarterly*, 8: 25–46.

Learman, L.A., Kupperman, M., Gates, E., Nease, R.F., Gildengorin, V. and Washington, A.E. (2003) 'Social and familial context of prenatal genetic testing decisions: are there racial/ethnic differences?' *American Journal of Medical Genetics (Part C)*, 119C: 190–26.

Lee, J. and Schmied, V. (2001) 'Involving men in antenatal education', *British Journal of Midwifery*, (9)9: 559–61.

Leshin, L. (2007) *Prenatal Screening for Down Syndrome* www.ds-health.com/prenatal.htm (accessed 2010).

Levy, V. (1999) 'Protective steering: a grounded theory study of the processes by which midwives facilitate informed choices during pregnancy', *Journal of Advanced Nursing*, 29(1): 104–12.

Lewando-Hundt, G., Shoham-Vardi, I., Beckerleg, S., Belmaker, I., Kassem, F. and Jaafar, A. (2001) 'Knowledge, Action and Resistance; the Selective Use of Pre-natal Screening among Bedouin Women of the Negev, Israel', *Social Science and Medicine*, 52(4): 561–9.

Lewis, S. (2001) 'Restructuring the workplace cultures: the ultimate work-family challenge?' *Women in Management Review*, 16(1): 21–29.

Locock, L. and Alexander, J. (2006) '"Just a bystander?" Men's place in the process of fetal screening and diagnosis', *Social Science and Medicine*, 62(6): 1349–59.

Lorber, J. (1989) 'Choice, gift or patriarchal bargain? Women's consent to invitro fertilization in male infertility', *Hypatia*, 4: 23.

Lorber, J. (1994) *Paradoxes of Gender*, New Haven and London: Yale University Press.

Lorber, J. and Bandlamudi, L. (1993) 'The dynamics of marital bargaining in male infertility', *Gender and Society*, 7(1): 32–49.

Lowe, P., Powell, J., Griffiths, F., Thorogood, M. and Locock, L. (2009) '"Making it all normal": the role of the Internet in problematic pregnancy', *Qualitative Health Research*, 19(10): 1476–84.

Lupton, D. and Barclay, L. (1997) *Constructing Fatherhood: Discourses and Experiences*, London: Sage.

Markens, S., Browner, C.H. and Preloran, H.M. (2003) '"I'm not the one they're sticking the needle into": Latino couples, fetal diagnosis, and the discourse of reproductive rights', *Gender and Society*, 17(3): 462–81.

Markens, S., Browner, C.H. and Press, N. (1997) 'Feeding the fetus: on interrogating the notion of maternal-fetal conflict', *Feminist Studies*, 23(2): 351–72.

Marshall, K. and Woollett, A. (2000) 'Fit to reproduce? The regulative role of pregnancy texts', *Feminism and Psychology*, 10(3): 351–66.

Marteau, T.M. and Dormandy, E. (2001) 'Facilitating informed choice in prenatal testing: how well are we doing?' *American Journal of Medical Genetics*, 106(3): 185–90.

Mason, D. (2003) *Explaining Ethnic Differences*, Bristol: Policy Press.

Matisons, M.R. (1997) 'The new feminist philosophy of the body' *The European Journal of Women's Studies*, 5: 9–34.

McCourt, C. (2006) 'Supporting choice and control? Communication and interaction between midwives and women at the antenatal booking visit', *Social Science and Medicine*, 62: 1307–18.

McLaughlin, J. (2003) 'Screening networks: shared agendas in feminist and disability movement challenges to antenatal screening and abortion', *Disability and Society*, 18 (3): 297–310.

Medhurst, A. (2000) 'If anywhere: class identification and cultural studies academics', in S.R. Munt (ed.), *Cultural Studies and the Working Class*, London: Cassell.

Meerabeau, L. (1991) 'Husbands' participation in fertility treatment. They also serve who stand and wait', *Sociology of Health and Illness*, 13: 396–410.

Mele, M.A. (2009) 'Exploring the gendered web', *Gender and Technology, Berkman Center for Internet and Society*, http://blogs.law.harvard.edu/genderandtech/tag/facebook/ (accessed May 2011).

Mitchell, L.M. and Georgies, E. (1997) 'Cross-cultural cyborgs: Greek and Canadian women's discourses on fetal ultrasound', *Feminist Studies*, 23(2): 373–401.

Modell, B., Harris, R., Lane, B., Khan, M., Darlison, M., Petrou, M., Old, J., Layton, M. and Varnavides, L. (2000) 'Informed choice in genetic screening for thalassaemia during pregnancy: audit from a national confidential inquiry', *British Medical Journal*, 320: 337–41.

Moyer, A., Brown, B., Gates, E., Daniels, M., Brown, H.D. and Kupperman, M. (1999) 'Decisions about prenatal testing for chromosomal disorders: perceptions of a diverse group of pregnant women', *Journal of Women's Health and Gender Based Medicine,* 8(4): 521–31.

Murkoff, H.E. and Mazel, S. (2009) *What to Expect When You Are Expecting?* London: Simon and Schuster.

Murphy, F. and Hunt, S. (1997) 'Early pregnancy loss: men have feelings too', *British Journal of Midwifery*, 5(2): 87–90.

Murray, J., Cuckle, H., Sehmi, I., Wilson, C. and Ellis, A. (2001) 'Quality of written information used in Down syndrome screening', *Prenatal Diagnosis*, 21: 138–42.

National Childbirth Trust (NCT) www.nct.org.uk/home (accessed February 2011).

National Institute of Neurological Disorders and Stroke, NINDS Microcephaly Information Page, www.ninds.nih.gov/disorders/microcephaly/microcephaly.htm (accessed 2011).

Nazroo, J. (2003) 'The structuring of ethnic inequalities in health: economic position, racial discrimination, and racism', *American Journal of Public Health*, 93(2): 277–84.

Net Mums www.netmums.com/ (accessed February 2011).

Nettleton, S. (1995) *Sociology of Health and Illness*, Cambridge: Polity Press.

NHS Choices (2008) 'Antenatal screening', www.nhs.uk/Conditions/Antenatal-screening (accessed 2008).

NHS Choices (2011) 'Miscarriage', www.nhs.uk/Conditions/Miscarriage/Pages/Introduction.aspx (accessed June 2011).

NHS Antenatal and Newborn Screening Programme (2008a) 'Sickle cell and thalassaemia' www.sct.screening.nhs.uk/Documents/MidwivesInfo.pdf (accessed 2008).

NHS Antenatal and Newborn Screening Programmes (2010) *Screening Tests for You and Your Baby*, NSC: UK National Screening Committee.

NHS Down's Syndrome Prevention (2008) www.nhsdirect.com (accessed 2008).

NHS Evidence (2011a) '(a)-Genetic conditions, Down's syndrome', www.library.nhs.uk/geneticconditions/viewresource.aspx?resID=88948 (accessed 2011).

NHS Evidence (2011b) '(b)-Genetic conditions, sickle cell anaemia', www.library.nhs.uk/geneticconditions/viewresource.aspx?resID=143175 (accessed 2011).

NHS Executive (2001) 'Good practice in consent: achieving the NHS plan commitment to patient-centred consent practice', www.dh.gov.uk/en/Publicationsandstatistics/Lettersandcirculars/Healthservicecirculars/DH_4003736 (accessed June 2011).

NICE (2003a) *Antenatal Care: Routine Care for the Healthy Pregnant Woman: Clinical Guidance*, National Collaborating Centre for Women's and Children's Health, London: RCOG Press.

NICE (2003b) *Routine Antenatal Care for Healthy Pregnant Women: Understanding NICE Guidance Information for Pregnant Women, Their Families and the Public*, London: NICE.

Nolan, J. and Scott, J. (2006) 'Gender and kinship networks in contemporary Britain', in M, Richards (ed.), *Kinship Relationships and Law in a Changing Society*, London: Hart.

Oakley, A. (1981) 'Interviewing women: a contradiction in terms', in Roberts, H. (ed), *Doing Feminist Research*, London: Routledge.

Oakley, A. (2005) (ed.) *The Ann Oakley Reader: Gender Women and Social Science*, Bristol: Policy Press.

OECD (2005) *Employment Outlook 2005*, Paris: OECD.

Olsson, P. and Jansson, L. (2001) 'Patterns in midwives and expectant/new parents ways of relating to each other in ante- and postnatal consultations', *Scandinavian Journal of Caring Sciences*, 15(2): 113–22.

Overall, C.H. (1987) *Ethics and Human Reproduction: A Feminist Analysis*, London: Allen & Unwin.

Pakulski, J. and Waters, M. (1996) *The Death of Class*, London: Sage.

Panter-Brick, C. (1991) 'Parental responses to consanguinity and genetic disease in Saudi Arabia', *Social Science and Medicine*, 33(11): 1295–302.

Petchesky, R. (1980) 'Reproductive freedom: beyond a women's right to choose', *Signs: Journal of Women in Culture and Society*, 5: 661–85.

Petchesky, R. (1984) *Abortion and Woman's Choice: The State, Sexuality and Reproductive Freedom*, Boston, MA: Northeastern University Press.

Petchesky, R. (1987) 'Foetal images: the power of visual culture in the politics of reproduction', in M. Stanworth (ed.), *Reproductive Technologies, Gender, Motherhood and Medicine*, Cambridge: Polity Press.

Pilnick, A. (2002) *Genetics and Society: An Introduction*, Buckingham: Open University Press.

Pilnick, A. (2004) '"It's just one of the best tests that we've got at the moment": the presentation of nuchal translucency screening for fetal abnormality in pregnancy', *Discourse and Society*, 15(4): 451–65.

Pizzini, F. (1992) 'Women's time, institutional time', in R. Frankenberg (ed), *Time, Health and Medicine*, London: Sage.

Plantin, L. (2001) *Men's Parenthood: On Men's Perceptions and Experiences of Fatherhood, (dissertation)*, Göteborg, University of Göteborg, Department of Social Work.

Plantin, L., Månsson, S.-A. and Kearney, J. (2003) 'Talking and doing fatherhood. On fatherhood and masculinity in Sweden and Britain', *Fathering*, 1: 3–26.

Pleck, J.H. (1987) 'American fathering in historical perspective', in M.S Kimmel (ed.), *Changing Men; New Research on Men and Masculinity*, London: Sage.

Press, N. and Browner, C. (1993) '"Collective fictions": similarities in reasons for accepting maternal serum alpha-fetoprotein screening among women of diverse ethnic and social class backgrounds,' *Fetal Diagnosis and Therapy*, 8(1): 97–106.

Press, N.A. and Browner, C.H. (1994) 'Collective silences, collective frictions: how prenatal diagnostic testing became part of routine prenatal care', in K.H. Rothenburg and E.J. Thompson (eds), *Women and Prenatal Testing: Facing the Challenges of Genetic Technology*, Ohio: Ohio State University Press.

Press, N. and Browner, C.H. (1997) 'Why women say yes to prenatal diagnosis', *Social Science and Medicine*, 45(7): 979–89.

Puthussery, S., Twamley, K., Harding, S., Mirsky, J., Baron, M. and Macfarlane, A. (2008) '"They're more like ordinary stroppy British women": attitudes and expectations of maternity care professionals to UK-born ethnic minority women', *Journal of Health Services Research and Policy*, 13(4): 195–201.

Rapp, R. (1994) 'Woman's responses to prenatal diagnosis: A sociocultural perspective on diversity', in K. Rothenberg and E. Thomson (eds), *Women and Prenatal Testing*, Columbus, OH: Ohio State University Press.

Rapp, R. (1998) 'Refusing prenatal diagnosis: the meanings of bioscience in a multicultural world', *Science and Technology Studies*, 23(1): 45–70.

Rapp, R. (2000) *Testing Women, Testing the Fetus*, London: Routledge.

Reed, K. (2003) *Worlds of Health*, Connecticut, USA: Praeger.

Reed, K. (2006) *New Directions in Social Theory: Race, Gender and the Canon*, London: Sage.

Reed, K. (2007a) 'Bureaucracy and beyond: the impact of ethical review and research governance on health research in the social sciences', *Sociological Research Online*, 12(5). www.socresonline.org.uk/12/5/18.html

Reed, K. (2007b) 'Antenatal screening and the gendering of genetic responsibility', *Reproductive Health*, 4:8. www.reproductive-health-journal.com/content/4/1/8

Reed, K. (2009a) '"It's them faulty genes again": women, men and the gendered nature of genetic responsibility', *Sociology of Health and Illness*, 31(3): 343–59.

Reed, K. (2009b) 'Fathers' involvement in antenatal screening: midwives' views', *British Journal of Midwifery*, 17(4): 218–22.

Reed, K. (2011a) 'Making men matter: exploring gender roles in prenatal screening', *Journal of Gender Studies*, 20(1): 55–66.

Reed, K. (2011b) '"He's the dad isn't he?" Gender, race and the politics of prenatal screening', *Ethnicity and Health* (Special Issue on Sickle Cell Disorders), 16 (4/5): 327–34.

Reitmanova, S. and Gustafson, D. (2008) '"They can't understand it": maternity health and care needs of immigrant Muslim women in St. John's, Newfoundland', *Maternal Child Health Journal*, 12(1): 101–11.

Richards, M. (1996) 'Families, kinship and genetics', in T. Marteau and M. Richards (eds), *The Troubled Helix: Social and Psychological Implications of the New Human Genetics*, Cambridge: Cambridge University Press.

Richardson, D. (2008) 'Conceptualizing gender', in D. Richardson and V. Robinson (eds), *Introducing Women's Studies: Feminist Theory and Practice*, 3rd edn, Basingstoke: Palgrave.

Ringrose, J. and Epstein, D. (2008) 'Gender and schooling: contemporary issues in gender equality and educational achievement', in D. Richardson and V. Robinson (eds), *Introducing Women's Studies: Feminist Theory and Practice*, 3rd edn, Basingstoke: Palgrave.

Rhodes, P.J. (1994) 'Race of interviewer effects: a brief comment', *Sociology*, 28: 547–58.

Robinson, V. (2008) 'Men, masculinities and feminism', in D. Richardson and V. Robinson (eds) *Introducing Women's Studies: Feminist Theory and Practice*, 3rd edn, Basingstoke: Palgrave.

Rose, H. (1987) 'Victorian values in a test-tube: the politics of reproductive science and technology', in M. Stanworth (ed.), *Reproductive Technologies: Gender, Motherhood and Medicine*, Cambridge: Polity.

Rose, N. (2001) 'The politics of life itself', *Theory, Culture and Society*, 18(6): 1–30.

Rothman, B.K. (1986) *The Tentative Pregnancy: How Amniocentesis Changes the Experience of Motherhood,* New York: Norton.

Rothman, B.K. (1995) 'Of maps and imaginations: sociology confronts the genome', *Social Problems*, 42: 1–10.

Rowe, R. and Garcia, J. (2005) 'Ethnic minorities' access to antenatal screening', *British Journal of Midwifery*, 13(2): 101–4.

Rowe, R.E. and Garcia, J. (2003) 'Social class, ethnicity and attendance for antenatal care in the United Kingdom: a systematic review', *Journal of Public Health Medicine*, 25(2): 113–19.

Rowe, R., Puddicombe, D., Hockley, C. and Redshaw, M. (2008) 'Offer and uptake of prenatal screening for Down syndrome in women from different social and ethnic backgrounds', *Prenatal Diagnosis*, 28(13): 1245–50.

Royal College of General Practitioners (2005) *Emma's Diary*, London: Lifecycle Marketing. Also www.emmasdiary.co.uk/ (accessed February 2011).

Sandelowski, M. (1994) 'Separate but less unequal: fetal ultrasonography and the transformation of expectant mother/fatherhood', *Gender and Society*, 8: 230–45.

Santalahti, P., Hemminki, E., Latikka, A. and Ryynanen, M. (1998) 'Women's decision-making in prenatal screening', *Social Science and Medicine*, 46(8): 1067–76.

Scheibal, F. and Dex, S. (1998) 'Should we have more family-friendly policies?' *European Management Journal*, 16(5): 586–99.

Schott, J. and Henley, A. (1997) *Culture, Religion and Childbearing in a Multiracial Society: A Handbook for Health Professionals*, Oxford: Butterworth-Heinemann.

Schuth, W., Karck, U., Wilhelm, C. and Reisch, S. (1994) 'Parents needs after ultrasound diagnosis of fetal malformation: an empirical deficit analysis', *Ultrasound in Obstetrics and Gynecology*, 124–9.

Scott, J. (2006) 'Family and gender roles: how attitudes are changing', *GenNet working paper*, No. 21, www.genet.ac.uk (accessed March 2009).

Scott, J. (2000) 'If class is dead, why won't it lie down?' In A. Woodward and G. Lengyel (eds), *European Societies: Inclusions and Exclusions*, London: Routledge.

Segal, L. (1990) *Slow Motion: Changing Masculinities, Changing Men*, New Brunswick, NJ: Rutgers University.

Simmonds, W. (2002) 'Watching the clock: keeping time in pregnancy, birth and post-partum experiences', *Social Science and Medicine*, 55(4): 559–70.

Shakespeare, T. (1995) 'Back to the future? New genetics and disabled people', *Critical Social Policy*, 44(5): 22–35.

Shakespeare, T. (1999) '"Losing the plot?" Medical and activist discourses of contemporary genetics and disability', *Sociology of Health and Illness*, 21(5): 669–88.

Shakespeare, T. (2008) 'Are we really more accepting of Down's syndrome?' guardian.co.uk (24/11/2008), www.guardian.co.uk/commentisfree/2008/nov/24/disability-children/print (accessed June 2011).

Smith, F.W., Adam, A.H. and Philips, W.D.P. (1983) 'NMR imaging in pregnancy', *Lancet*, 321(8314–15): 61–2.

Skeggs, B. (1997) *Formations of Class and Gender: Becoming Respectable*, London: Sage.

Skeggs, B. (2001) 'The toilet paper: femininity, class, and mis-recognition', *Women's Studies International Forum*, 24(3/4): 295–307.

Stanworth, M. (1987) (ed.) *Reproductive Technologies: Gender, Motherhood and Medicine*, Polity: Cambridge.

Steinberg, D.L. (1997) *Bodies in Glass: Genetics, Eugenics, Embryo Ethics*, Manchester: Manchester University Press.

Stenson, K., Sidenvall, B. and Heimer, G. (2005) 'Midwives' experiences of routine antenatal questioning relating to men's violence against women', *Midwifery*, 21(4): 311–21.

Streetly, A., Latinovic, R. and Henthorn, J. (2010) 'Positive screening and carrier results for the England-wide universal newborn sickle cell screening programme by ethnicity and area for 2005–7', *Journal of Clinical Pathology*, 63: 626–9.

Sullivan, J.R. (1999) 'Development of father-infant attachment in fathers of preterm infants', *Neonatal Network*, 18: 33–9.

Tsianakas, V. and Laimputtong, P. (2002) 'What women from an Islamic background in Australia say about care in pregnancy and prenatal testing', *Midwifery*, 18(1): 25–34.

UK National Screening Committee (2003) 'Antenatal screening – working standards incorporating those for the National Down Syndrome screening programme for England', January 2003, www.nelh.nhs.uk/screening/dssp/Standards.pdf (accessed 2008).

UK National Screening Committee (2007) 'Antenatal screening – working standards for Down's syndrome screening', www.perinatal.nhs.uk/ultrasound/screening/WorkingStandardsforDownsSyndromeScreening%202007.pdf (accessed June 2011).

Van Allen, M.I. and Myhre, S. (1991) 'New multiple congenital anomalies syndrome in a stillborn infant of consanguinous parents and a prediabetic pregnancy', *American Journal of Medical Genetics*, 38(4): 523–8.

Vosler, A.T. and Burst, H.V. (1993) 'Nurse-midwifery as it reinforces and transforms the American ideology of gendered roles', *Journal of Nurse-Midwifery*, 38(5): 293–300.

Wailoo, K. (2001) *Dying in the City of the Blues: Sickle Cell Anemia and the Politics of Race and Health*, NC: The University of North Carolina Press.

Wailoo, K. and Pemberton, S. (2006) *The Troubled Dream of Genetic Medicine*, Baltimore, MD: Johns Hopkins University Press.

Walby, S. (1990) *Theorizing Patriarchy*, Oxford: Blackwell.

Wall, G. and Arnold, S. (2007) 'How involved is involved fathering? An exploration of the contemporary culture of fatherhood', *Gender and Society*, 21: 508–27.

Webster, A. (2007) *Health, Technology and Society: A Sociological Critique*, Basingstoke: Palgrave Macmillan.

Whitby, E.H., Paley, M.N., Sprigg, A., Rutter, S., Davies, N.P., Wilkinson, I.D. and Griffiths, P.D. (2004) 'Comparison of ultrasound and magnetic resonance imaging in 100 singleton pregnancies with suspected brain abnormalities', *BJOG*, 111: 784–92.

Williams, C., Alderson, P. and Farisides, B. (2002) '"Too many choices?" Hospital and community staff reflect on the future of prenatal screening', *Social Science and Medicine*, 55: 743–53.
Williams, K. and Umberson, D. (1999) 'Medical technology and childbirth: experiences of expectant mothers and fathers', *Sex Roles*, 41(314): 147–68.
Witz, A. (2000) 'Whose body matters? Feminist sociology and the corporeal turn in sociology and feminism', *Body and Society*, 6(2): 1–24.
World Health Organization (2007) *Fatherhood and Health Outcomes in Europe: A Summary Report*, Denmark: WHO, regional office, www.euro.who.int/–data/assets/pdf_file/0019/69013/E91129sum.pdf (accessed June 2011).
Yoon, P.W., Scheuner, M.T., Peterson-Oehlke, K.L., Gwinn, M., Faucett, A. and Khoury, M.J. (2002) 'Can family history be used as a tool for public health and preventative medicine?' *Genetics in Medicine*, 4(4): 304–10.
Zechmeister, I. (2001) 'Foetal images: the power of visual technology in antenatal care and the implications for women's reproductive freedom', *Health Care Analysis*, 9(4): 387–400.

Index

Adam, B. 46, 48, 50
agency 41, 87

blood group 43, 65, 67–68, 76
Bourdieu, P. 142–43

capital: cultural 141, 143–45, 159; economic 143, 148–49; social 143
choice: diagnostic testing 43–46; genetics 15, 39, 57, 136; reproductive 40–42 *see also* reproductive autonomy; women and screening 42–43, 57, 164; time in screening 46–48; and male choice 52–54, 58, 164
Chorionic Villus Sampling (CVS) 11
Connell, R. 24, 38, 94,165, 168
combined testing *see* integrated testing
corporeality 15, 39, 164, 179

Delphy, C. 2, 6, 87
disability: choice 41; Down's syndrome 44, 106–7, 113, 122, 144; family 127, 131, 136; reproductive genetics 98, 100, 103, 109, 113; race and ethnicity 140, 150, 153, 160; *see also* Down's syndrome
DNA 3, 15, 64–65, 99, 107, 164
Down 's Syndrome: Down's Syndrome Association 106; definition of 9–10; public perceptions 106; types of screening and diagnostic testing 10–11
Dragonas, T. 100, 109, 112–13, 179
Dyson, S. 104, 135, 149

Edwards Syndrome, 10
Employment policy 177–78; *see also* work
Ettorre, E: maternal age 85, 99; gender 8; genetic capital 98, 112; women and genetics 15–16, 59, 64, 76, 97, 112–13, 164–65; women's roles in reproduction 3, 100, 114
Eugenics 96; race 96–97; screening and disability 97

family: extended family 127–28; female relatives 123–25; history and screening 16–17, 63, 75, 115–16, 118, 128–36; resemblance 74–76; screening 16, 115–17, 136, 165–66; women and men 125–27; women as mediators of 37
faulty genes 16, 105, 109–14, 165
femininity 7, 8, 80
Finger, A. 16, 97–98, 101, 106, 113

gender paradox 19, 38, 163, 165, 168
gender role ideology 7, 8, 162, 179; institutions of 8, 163, 166, 168
genetic capital 98, 102, 111–12, 114, 139; identity 98; potential 98, 100, 111, 114
Giddens, A. 30, 46, 132, 136, 138, 167

Haraway, D. 70
hereditary illness 101, 129–30
Hochschild, A. 55–56, 58, 168
Human Genome Project 96

inequality 17, 98, 138–39, 159–61, 166, 168; gender 7–8, 167–68; social class 141–42; *see also* race and ethnicity, and social class
information: gender and screening 14, 24–27, 164; health professionals and 29–30; improving men's access to 171; pregnancy related 18–21; women and 21–23; women as gatekeepers of 21, 24, 27–29; *see also* the Internet
integrated testing 10
internet: health and pregnancy 41–42; men and 14–15, 19, 21, 33–35, 38, 164; problematic pregnancies 20, 35–36; women and 20, 32–33, 37–38

Jordan, P.L. 4, 7, 78

Kerr, A. 15, 39–41, 57, 97, 138
kinship 108, 115, 118–19, 127–29, 131–34; definition of 122–23; medicalisation of 128, 136

LaRossa, R. 4–5, 58, 79, 88
Lorber, J: gender change 180; gender ideology 58; gender paradox 163; gendered institutions 8, 168; male breadwinner 5, 7; women and pregnancy 69

masculinity: decision-making 79–80; diverse nature of 167–68; hegemonic 38, 94, 165, 168; theoretical framework 7–8; traditional 24, 36, 38; *see also* new fatherhood
maternity 3, 53, 64–65, 69, 99, 150, 172
microcephaly 103; 109–12, 114, 130–31
milestones 39; of pregnancy 48–50, 58
miscarriage: diagnostic testing11, 84–85, 89, 91, 117, 127; in early pregnancy 49
MRI 10–11, 60

NRTs (New Reproductive Technology) 3, 178
Nuchal fold (or translucency) scan 10, 16, 46–48, 59–60, 81, 90–91; friends 105, 119–20; social class 144–45, 148, 159
new fatherhood 4–5, 16, 78–79, 94, 165; cultural shift of 2, 4–5, 78; decision-making 81–83; information 38

paternity 67, 74, 77; patriarchy 3, 64, 99, 165; pay and leave 56, 178; *see also* patriarchy
patriarchy 3, 64, 99, 169; *see also* Walby, S.
Pilnick, A: blood disorders 104; eugenics 96; kinship 122–23, 128, 139; screening and testing 8, 10–11; ultrasound and diagnostic testing 60, 89

race and ethnicity: concepts of 151; gender 156–59; genetic conditions 149; prenatal screening 139–41, 149–51, 159–60; serum screening 1 53–54; *see also* whiteness
racial discrimination 140, 150, 152, 160
racialisation 135, 141, 151, 156, 160
Rapp, R: amniocentesis 43, 51, 76; class and race 139–41, 143–45, 148, 150, 153, 156, 159; gender and screening 17, 34, 94, 163; genetics 3, 99; male control 86, 93; pregnancy and women 6, 76, 174; kinship and disability 115–17, 127, 131, 136; women and reproductive responsibility 26, 78–79, 99, 100, 114; women as fetal guardians 3, 18, 20, 28
regulation 18, 20, 31
reproductive autonomy 3–4, 28–29, 163, 175–78; decision-making 78–79, 81, 87, 165; health professionals 94–95, 176–77; information 37–38; screening policy 29, 92
risk society 138
Rh disease 67
Rose, N. 15, 39–40, 136, 138
Rothman, B. K. 99–101, 103, 106, 112, 165; choice 41; decision-making 78, 84, 87; disability 85; eugenics 97; patriarchy 3, 64, 67, 77; testing 15–16

Sandelowski, M: male inseminator role 3, 69, 74, 173; parent centred maternity care 68–69; ultrasound and men's involvement 6–7, 15, 59, 69, 73–74, 164; women, men and pregnancy 2–3; *see also* ultrasound
Segal, L. 80
Shakespeare, T. 41, 97, 106
Sickle cell disease: antenatal screening 9; definition of 9
social class: definition of 142–43; measures of 141; screening 17, 78, 139–41, 143–45, 159–61, 166; youth 145–47; work 58, 147–49; *see also* work
Sonocaid 62, 66, 71; doppler fetal monitor 70; ultrasound transducer 62, 66, 70, 72, 76; *see also* ultrasound
space: men and reproduction 3, 36, 69, 74, 173; social 142; women 15, 39, 48; *see also* time
Spina Bifida 49, 62, 99, 106–8, 110, 149; high risk pregnancy 35, 88–89; screening for 10

Thalassaemia: antenatal screening for 9; definition of 9
time: men 15, 54–58, 164; professional 50–52; reproduction 39; screening 15, 46–48, 57, 164; space 3; symbolic 48; *see also* milestones, and space
Turners Syndrome 10, 97

ultrasound scan: gender and 68–70, 76; its use 10–11; men and 15, 72–75, 76–77, 164; the importance of visual technology 60–62

Webster 138–39, 141–42, 161
whiteness 141, 151, 160; gender roles 157–58; haemoglobinopathy screening 154–56, 160, 166
work: family friendly work policies 54, 178; gendered model of 56; genetic screening in the workplace 138–39; male model of 55, 58; workplace norms 5, 15, 40, 55, 164, 176